IMAGES
of America

NAPA STATE HOSPITAL

On the Cover: This postcard photograph titled "Through the gateway—State Hospital Napa, Calif." It represents the paradox of mental health issues to most people. It is visible and present in everyday life; however, a full understanding of the complexities of caring for patients is elusive, especially to their caretakers. (Courtesy Todd Schulman.)

IMAGES
of America

NAPA STATE HOSPITAL

Patricia Prestinary
Foreword by Lauren Coodley

ARCADIA
PUBLISHING

ISBN 978-1-4671-3199-5

Published by Arcadia Publishing
Charleston, South Carolina

Printed in the United States of America

Library of Congress Control Number: 2013956260

For all general information, please contact Arcadia Publishing:
Telephone 843-853-2070
Fax 843-853-0044
E-mail sales@arcadiapublishing.com
For customer service and orders:
Toll-Free 1-888-313-2665

Visit us on the Internet at www.arcadiapublishing.com

Contents

Foreword

Reading this book is like being handed the key to the door in the attic. Lingering inside that room are the images of the madwoman from Charlotte Brontë's *Jane Eyre*, from Frances Farmer's *Will There Really Be a Morning?*, and from Janet Frame's *Faces in the Water*. But, as we learn from the opening pages of this book, the Napa public was able to walk right into the asylum. The attendants and doctors lived on the grounds, and they stare back from the pages of this extraordinary volume.

The establishment of the Napa Asylum was part of a reform movement to create a sanctuary for those considered unacceptable in mainstream society. In the 19th century, mental illness was viewed as a character defect or hereditary problem. It was not seen as a medical problem, or at least not one that involved the need for medication. Joseph Amato tells us that patients in the early asylums "were sorted according to the period's primitive psychological structures, which merged prejudices, morality, philosophy, and the new science of psychology in odd combinations."

I began working at the state hospital in 1977. I was transfixed by the fragile women whom I met there, the kind of women whom we would now find at encampments in every major city in America. Back then, people with drug and alcohol problems as well as violent, depressed, and schizophrenic people were simply picked up and dropped off at the state hospital. I was surrounded by a plethora of skilled professionals: psychologists, nurses, social workers, and psychiatric technicians.

In the decades since, the hospital has emptied as a result of well-intentioned, if perhaps mistaken, legislation that tossed the mentally ill into board and care homes or onto the streets. The legislation did include some rights for patients in an effort to reduce abuse. The result, though, was an explosion of homelessness and the loss of economic security that employment at the hospital had offered thousands of Napans. Continue on in this book to learn about the history of mental illness as this institution changed over a period of 100 years, from 1875 to 1975, and to view—and imagine—the stories of those who lived there, both as patients and as their caretakers.

—Lauren Coodley

Acknowledgments

Special thanks to Nancy Levenberg and Alexandria Brown from the Napa County Historical Society. This book would not have been completed without the guidance and expertise of scholars Lauren Coodley and Ellen Brannick. I also owe a debt of gratitude to Napa State Hospital librarian Carl Seele and to the Department of State Hospitals. I would also like to thank the Napa residents and former employees who shared their stories and collections: Cindi Hummer, Patricia Renait, Todd Schulman, Laurence Seaton, Darrell Turner, Connie Wallace, and Peter Zwetsloot.

Courtesies for the images are abbreviated for the following organizations: California State Archives (CSA), Napa County Historical Society (NCHS), and Napa State Hospital (NSH).

Introduction

On April 18, 1872, Gov. Newton Booth appointed Dr. E.T. Wilkins of Marysville, Dr. Benjamin Shurtleff of Stockton, and Judge C.H. Swift of Sacramento as commissioners to select a Bay Area site for California's second asylum. The site was located two miles southeast of Napa, and on August 2, 1872, part of Rancho Tulocay, a total of 209 acres of land, was purchased from Don Cayetano Juarez for $11,506.

The asylum's first board of directors was composed of J.H. Jewett of Marysville, Dr. J.F. Morris of San Francisco, James H. Goodman of Napa, Chancellor Harlan, R.H. Stirling of Napa, Dr. John F. Morse, and W.C. Watson, whose first meeting was held in Napa with Drs. Wilkins and Shurtleff on September 13, 1872. Work on the massive building began in October 1872, and on January 23, 1873, San Francisco architects Wright & Sanders were selected to design an asylum for $600,000. Construction was a slow process and often halted until more funds could be obtained from the state legislature, which waged bitter battles in Sacramento over the "extravagant use of public funds." By the time the building was completed, it cost $1.75 million. The *Napa Register* responded to the scandal in defense of the building, calling it "the finest building in the State." It went on to state, "All jobs having been let on bids under severe competition, it is probably the cheapest building the State ever built." The cornerstone was laid with a ceremony on December 24, 1875.

Dr. Edwin Bentley of San Francisco was appointed as the first superintendent on October 18, 1874, then was replaced by Dr. E.T. Wilkins four months after the first patients arrived to the Napa Asylum for the Insane on November 15, 1875. Dr. Wilkins was a widely respected administrator and physician who contributed extensively to both the state and the asylum's early mental health efforts during his many years of service.

Expansion marked Supt. A.M. Gardner's term. Built between 1875 and 1930 were 19 staff and patient residences, eight maintenance and farm structures, and six dams, along with the paving of several roads and the construction of a bus shelter—all with patient labor and bricks made on-site. Cog rails were installed in the basement to transport laundry and food to each of the seven towers. By 1954, there were over 300 structures on the hospital grounds, including ward buildings, maintenance shops, farm structures, officers' homes, employees' residences, and garages. Additional property was purchased, and at its peak, it occupied over 2,000 acres.

Patients worked on the farming and maintenance operations, sewed clothing, crocheted, knitted, embroidered, wove baskets and colonial mats, and made items of brass, copper, and clay, which the hospital either used or sold. Occupational therapy, or moral treatment, guaranteed that the asylum was self-sufficient, and it continued well into 1966, when the Fair Labor Standards Act required that state hospitals begin paying patients for their labor. In 1977, occupational therapy was replaced by optional vocational services programs, which paid patients 30¢ to 60¢ per hour for work that was supplemental to the essential functioning of the facility.

In 1924, the Department of Institutions was established, and all California Asylums for the Insane were renamed to reflect changes in the medical community. The Napa Asylum for the Insane was thereafter called the Napa State Hospital.

After 75 years as a landmark in Napa, maintenance for "the Castle" became an encumbrance. A lack of modern facilities hindered patient care, which was already suffering due to overcrowding. Reports of overcrowding led Gov. Earl Warren to conduct surveys of the state hospitals in 1942. The grand architectural statement that was known as "the Castle" was declared a firetrap and slated for destruction. The state set aside $15 million for the demolition and replacement of the Castle; however, construction was delayed due to materials and labor shortage during the war. Supt. Theo K. Miller oversaw the transformation of the Napa State Hospital and was responsible for initiating the children's unit, the coordinated therapies program, and the clinical research program.

Gov. Goodwin J. Knight dedicated the new Receiving and Treatment Center on December 12, 1954. The updated treatment model, "total push," was reserved for acute patients and included work therapy, individual and group therapy, and social activities. It was designed to provide skills needed to reintegrate patients into their communities. Social services and day-care clinics were established at this time to provide support and services to patients on an outpatient basis.

Advances in psychotropic drug therapies and changing legislation introduced to protect the civil rights of the mentally ill and developmentally disabled reshaped the function of California state hospitals. Starting in 1967 with cutbacks ordered by Gov. Ronald Reagan and in 1968 with the Lanternman-Short-Petris Act, the process of deinstitutionalization began. Napa State Hospital closed its dairy, sold farmland to the Napa Valley College, Kennedy Park, and returned the land that is now part of Skyline Park to the State of California. These closures had a huge impact on Napa Valley, as the state hospital had been a major employer and home to hundreds of employees and their families.

One

The Castle
1875–1921

Controversy has always encircled those with mental illness and their caretakers. In the early 19th century, reformists such as Dorothea Dix sought to apply Enlightenment values and modern scientific methods to the treatment of the mentally ill. A movement sprang up throughout Europe and the United States that influenced practitioners such as Dr. Thomas Kirkbride, whose detailed plans for the construction and management of hospitals for the insane served as the blueprint for hundreds of institutions built in the United States in the mid to late 19th century.

Before Stockton Asylum was built in 1850, California's mentally ill patients were housed in a ship anchored in San Francisco Bay off of San Quentin Point. Using Stockton as a basis for comparison, Dr. Edmund T. Wilkins visited 149 institutions as part of a six-month survey of U.S. and European facilities and treatments. He had been commissioned by Gov. Raymond Haight to develop a plan and find a site for a new facility, which there was dire need for due to overcrowding in the Stockton Asylum. He chose the Kirkbride Plan and selected Napa because there were over 100 acres of arable land, in the country and yet close to a town, with a water supply and nearby wharf.

Napa Asylum for the Insane opened on November 15, 1875, with its first patient an alcoholic from San Francisco. In January 1876, sixty patients were transferred from Stockton Asylum. Proponents of "moral treatment" believed in the healing influence of the hospital and its environment. According to Nancy Tomes in *A Generous Confidence*, the aim of moral treatment was "to alleviate the psychological causes of mental disease by radically changing the individual's environment and daily regimen." The mission of Napa Asylum was, from the outset, to cure mental illness and prepare patients for the rigors of daily life. The magnificent structure and grounds were compared to European castles, and the town's namesake was taken from another scenic town with an asylum: Imola, Italy.

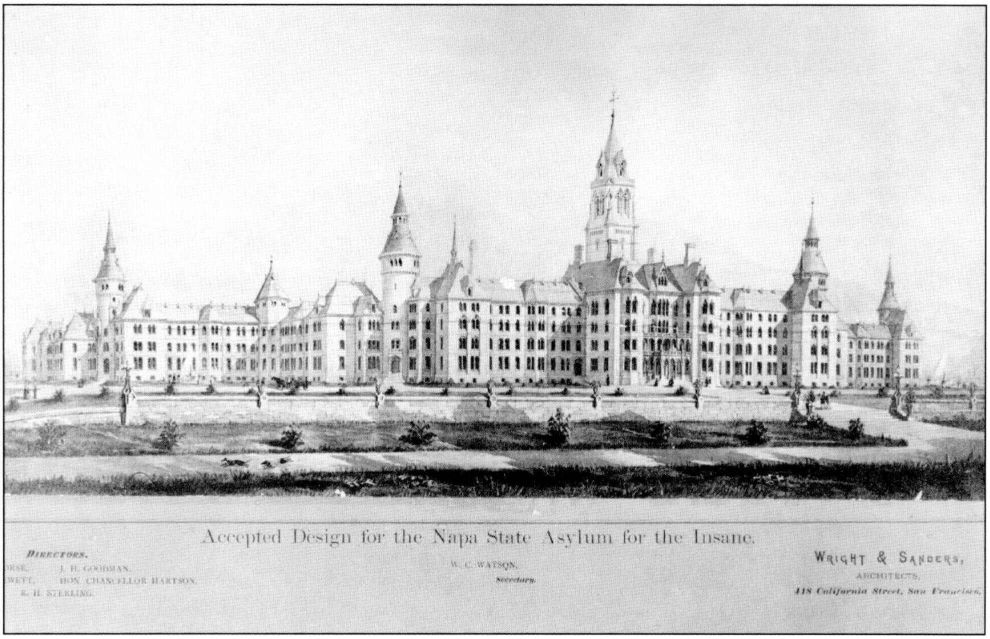
Accepted Design for the Napa State Asylum for the Insane.
Directors.
J. H. Goodman.
Hon. Chancellor Hartson.
W. C. Watson,
Secretary.
Wright & Sanders,
Architects,
418 California Street, San Francisco.

Gov. Raymond Haight commissioned Dr. Edmund T. Wilkins to conduct a study of other psychiatric hospitals due to overcrowding in the Stockton Asylum. Napa was selected as the location for California's second institution, and the state purchased 208 acres from Don Cayetano Juarez. San Francisco architects Wright & Saunders designed the facility. (Courtesy NCHS.)

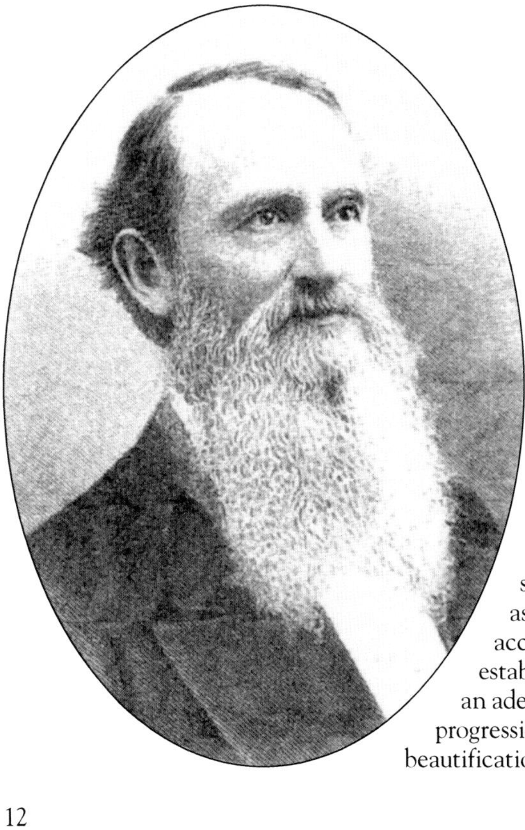

Dr. Edmund T. Wilkins studied 149 institutions in North America and Europe before recommending the "moral treatment" of the mentally ill. He was on the commission to select the location of the new facility and served as superintendent from 1876 to 1891. Among his accomplishments at the Napa Asylum were the establishment of a system of lakes and reservoirs for an adequate water supply, development of farmland, progression of positive community relationships, and beautification of the grounds. (Courtesy NSH.)

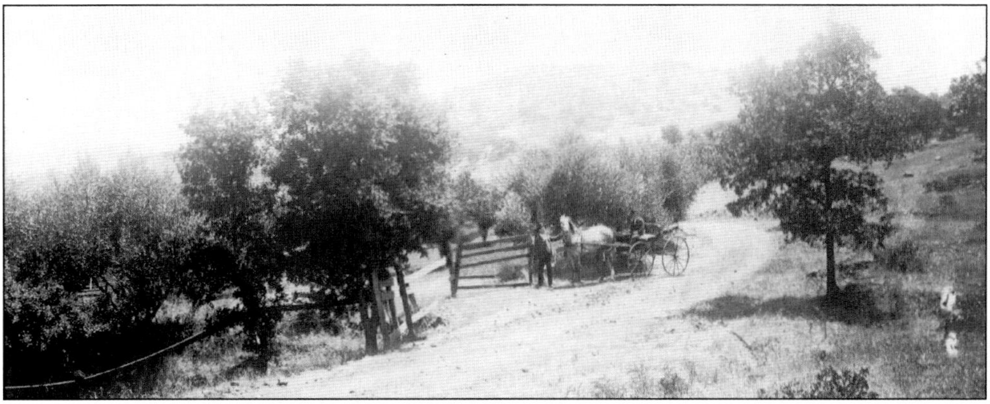

Napa was chosen as the site for the second California asylum because the land fulfilled the standards as set forth in Thomas Kirkbride's *On the Construction, Organization, and General Arrangements of Hospitals for the Insane*. With over 100 acres of arable land in the countryside, the site boasted attractive scenery and a supply of water in addition to its proximity to town (two miles), roads, and a railroad. It also was located near a wharf on the Napa River from which they could receive supplies. (Courtesy NCHS.)

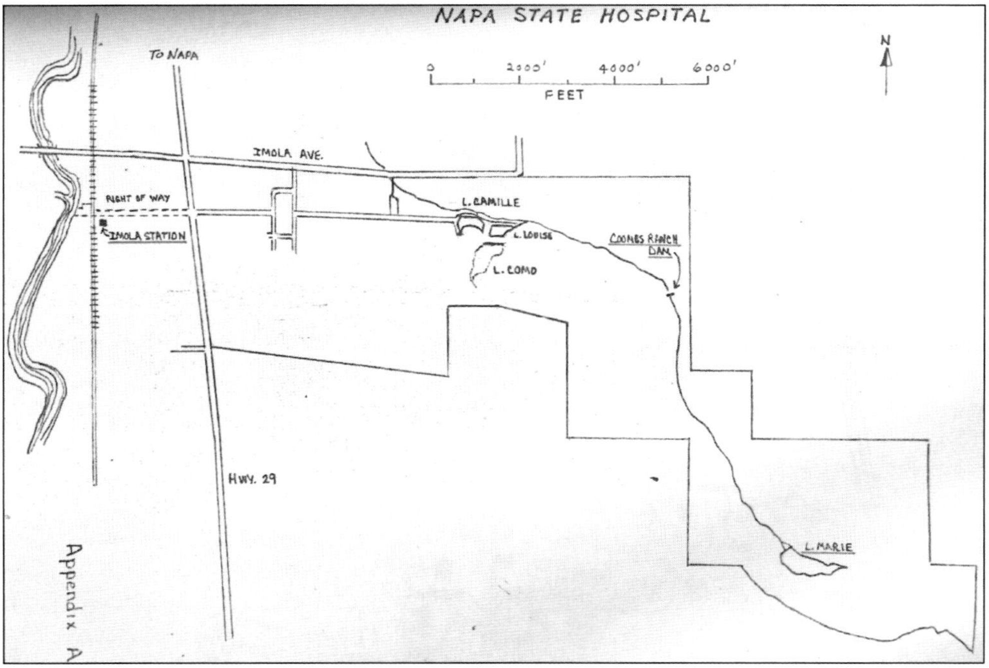

This map, extracted from the Historic Resources Inventory taken in 1980 by Napa State Hospital Historian Ellen Brannick, shows the locations of the three lakes, Coombs Dam, Imola Avenue, the Napa-Vallejo Highway (in the illustration as "Hwy 29"), and the Imola station. The small rectangle in the upper left shows the location of the Castle. Lake Marie, in the lower right, was the main supplier to the lower lakes. Located in the center of the map, adjacent to Lake Camille and Lake Louise, the Lake Como Dam was built in 1890 and is now a dry lake bed. It was the largest lower lake, with a capacity of 20 million gallons and an elevation of 160 feet. Its earthen dam functioned as a levee that formed on the north side of the reservoir, and the natural slope of the hills formed the other shorelines. A concrete spillway was found near the northeast end, and water spilled into Lake Louise. (Courtesy Napa City-County Library.)

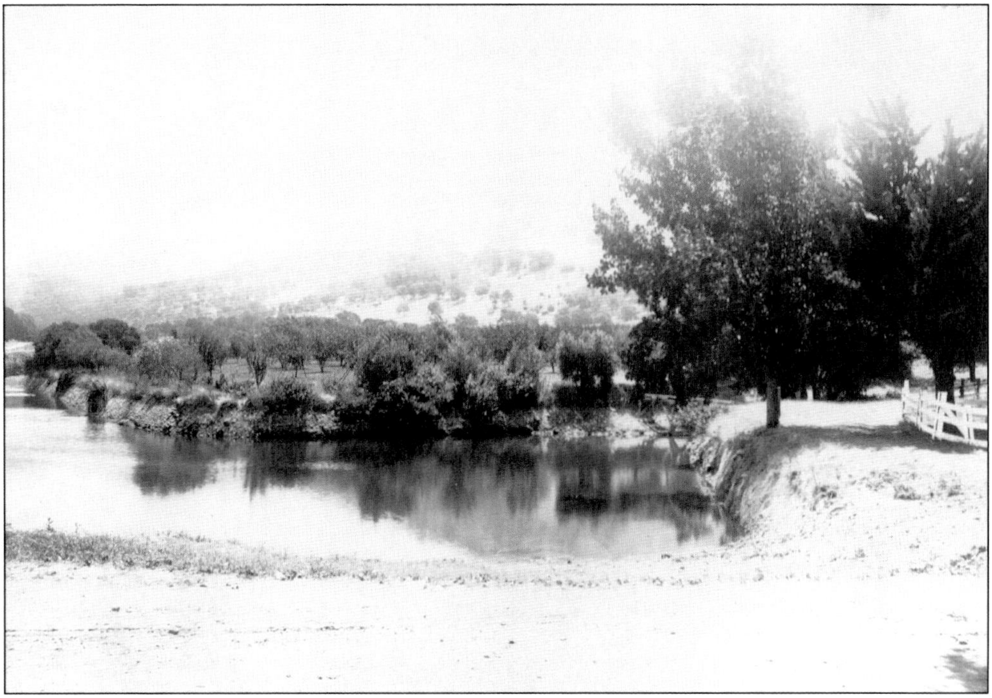

Lake Camilla, named after the wife of Dr. Wilkins, provided the first of three large lower-water reserves for irrigation, watering of livestock, and esthetic pleasure. It was intended to hold seven million gallons of water, but by its completion in 1885 it had been enlarged to 10 million gallons at an elevation of 125 feet to provide proper gravity flow to the grounds. In 1888, the reservoir was enlarged to 12 million gallons. Water entered from either Lake Louise or Lake Como, and an orchard was named Martha's Vineyard after the daughter of Dr. Wilkins. (Courtesy NCHS.)

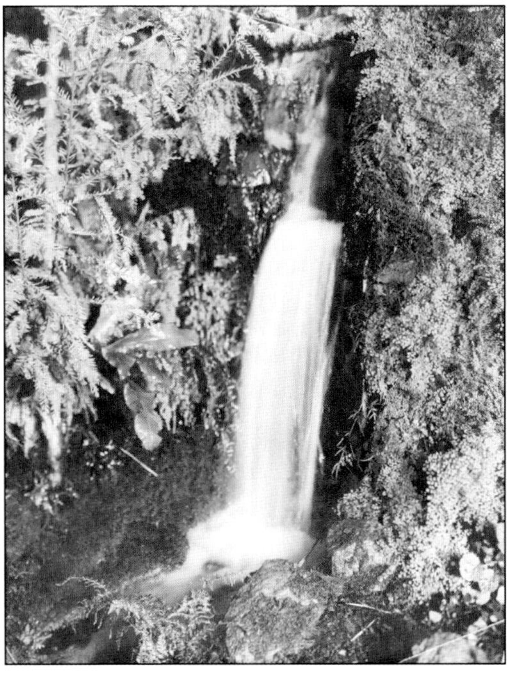

The Coombs Ranch Dam, one of the site's oldest structures, was built in 1872. It is 10 feet high, with a narrow floodgate set to the upper left center. Visitors and patients reached it by walking up a beautiful narrow path, past an old lathhouse, a fireplace, and rough stone walls built by patients. Pictured here is one of several waterfalls on the grounds. (Courtesy NSH.)

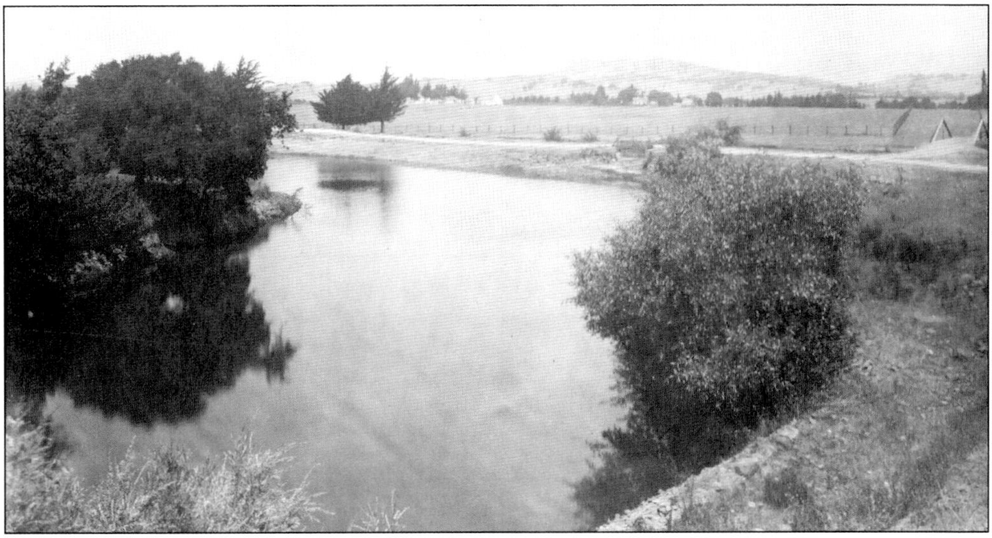

The original name for Lake Louise, a reservoir, was Lake Lucerne, but no reason has been found for the name change. At an elevation of 145 feet, it was the location of a second earthen dam completed in 1888. It was planned as a reservoir with a capacity of eight million gallons, but it was enlarged during construction to hold 10 million gallons. Water flowed in from south Tulocay Creek at the east end or a pipe from Lake Como. Excess water flowed over the concrete spillway on the north levee and into the creek or was directed through a pipe in the west bank to Lake Camille. The road on the levee leads to the east past orchard remains to the Camp Coombs area. A chicken ranch was located across the road on the north levee. (Courtesy NCHS.)

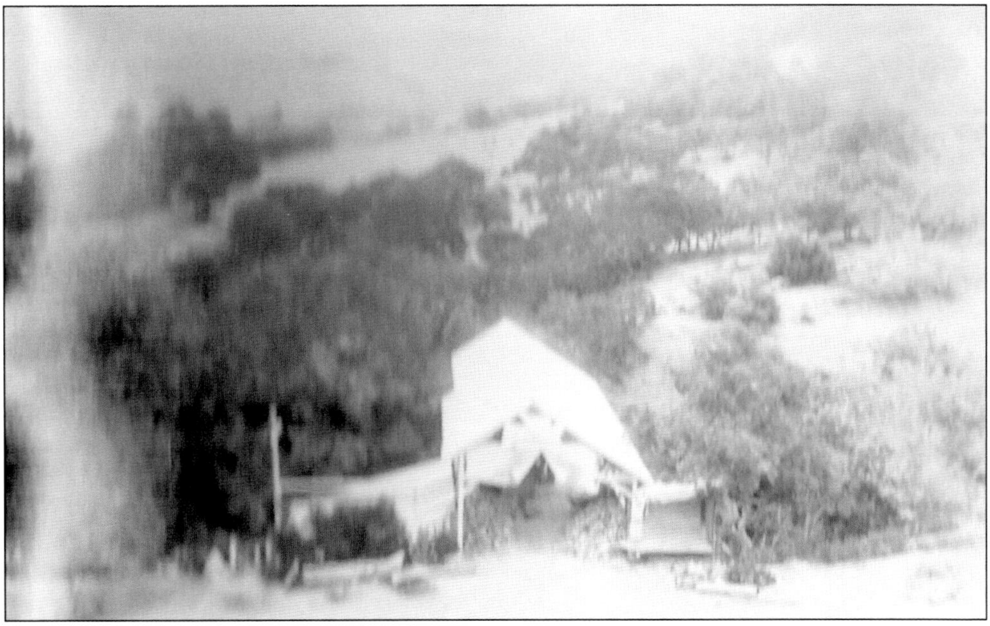

Stones from the property were used to construct the main building, several other structures, and roads. The on-site stone quarry was later leased to the Basalt Rock Company; the rock crusher pictured was likely part of the quarry. Founded in 1920, the Basalt Rock Company's products were used in the construction of Treasure Island, the site of the 1939 Golden Gate International Exposition, and they later branched out into steel fabrication. (Courtesy CSA.)

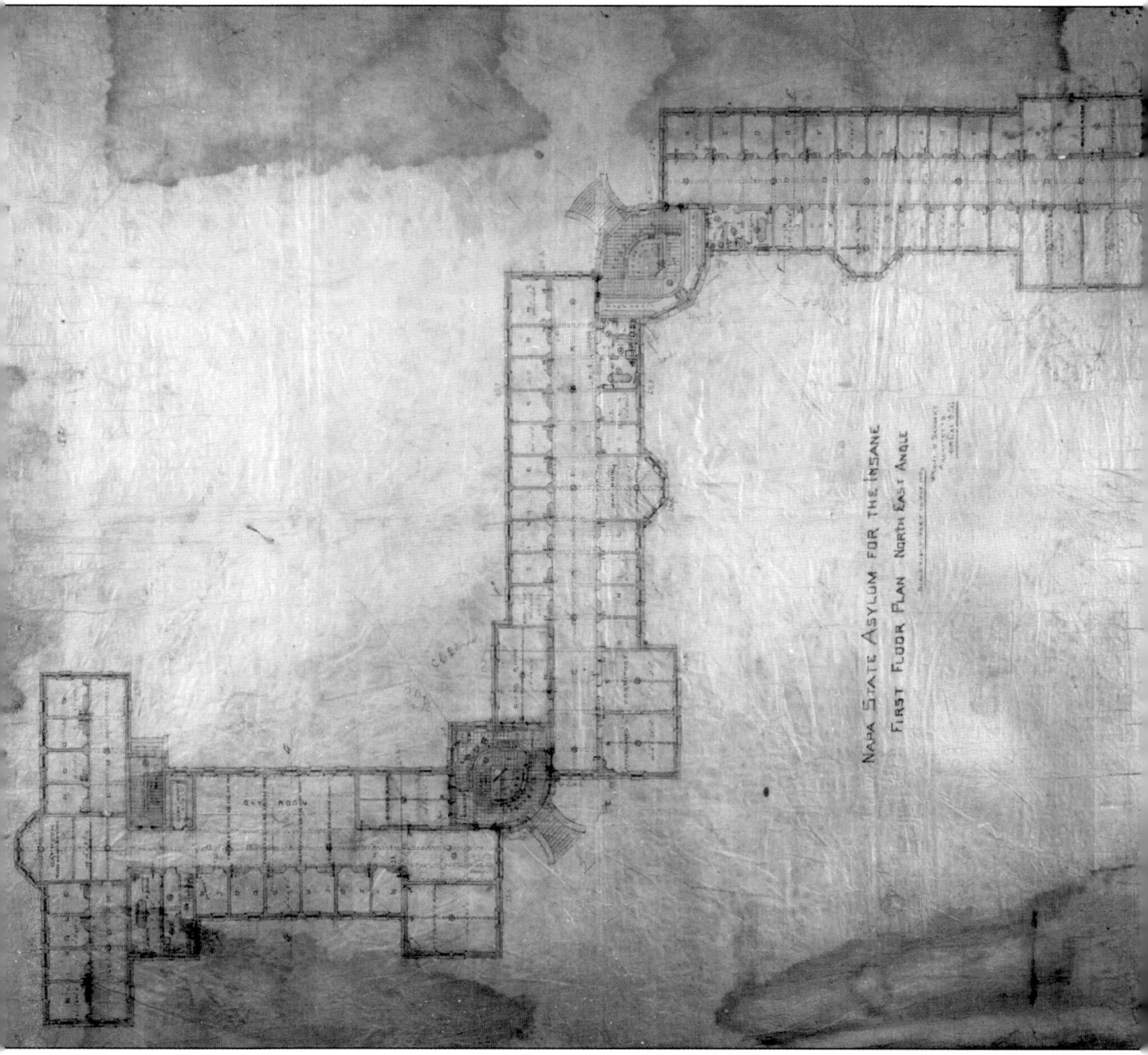

These blueprints were laid in the cornerstone during a ceremony on December 24, 1874. A mile in circumference, the Romantic Gothic building stood on 208 acres of land. Accommodations were

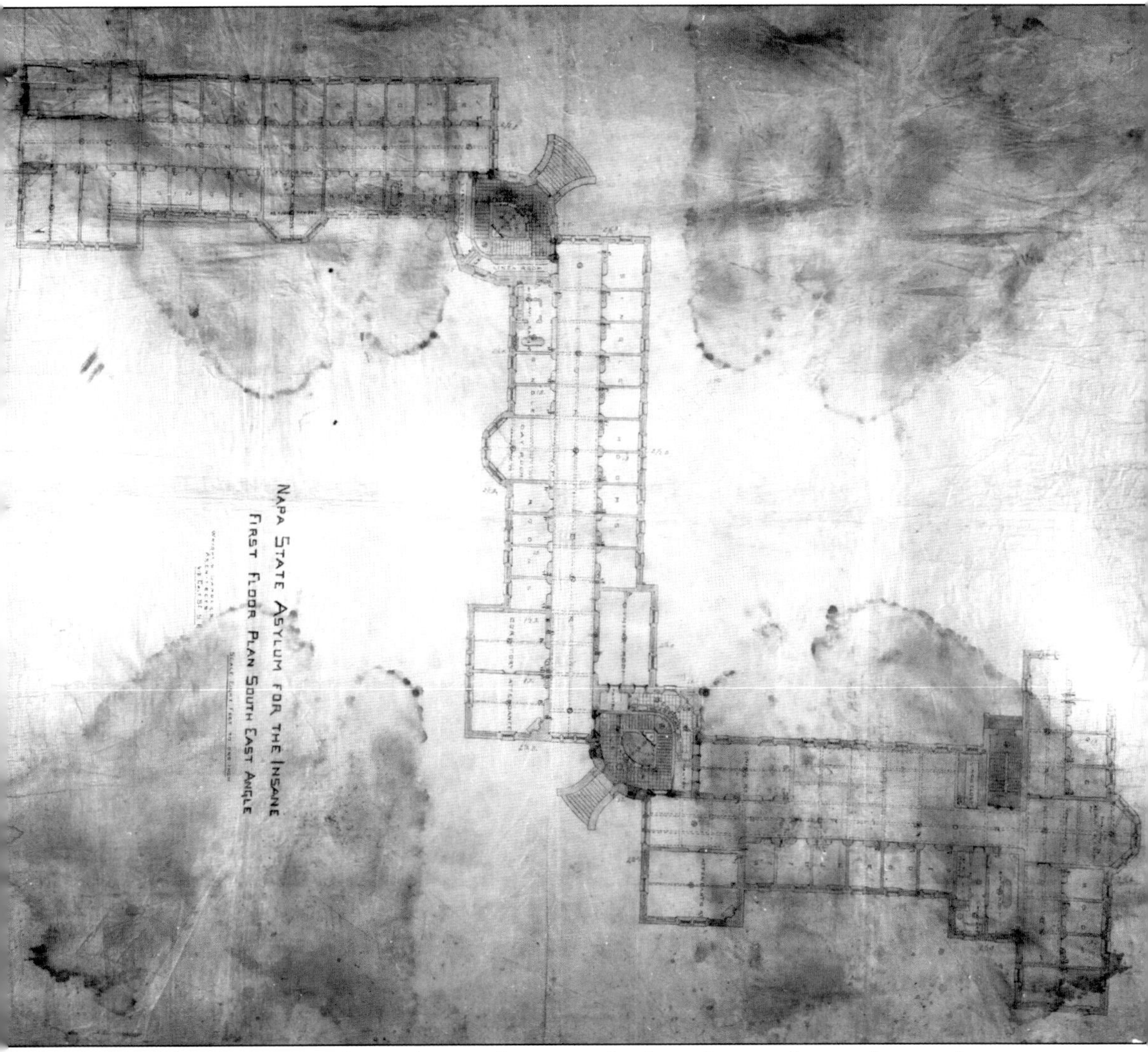

included for 640 patients. It was three to five stories high, with seven fireproof towers forming a continuous front line. (Courtesy CSA.)

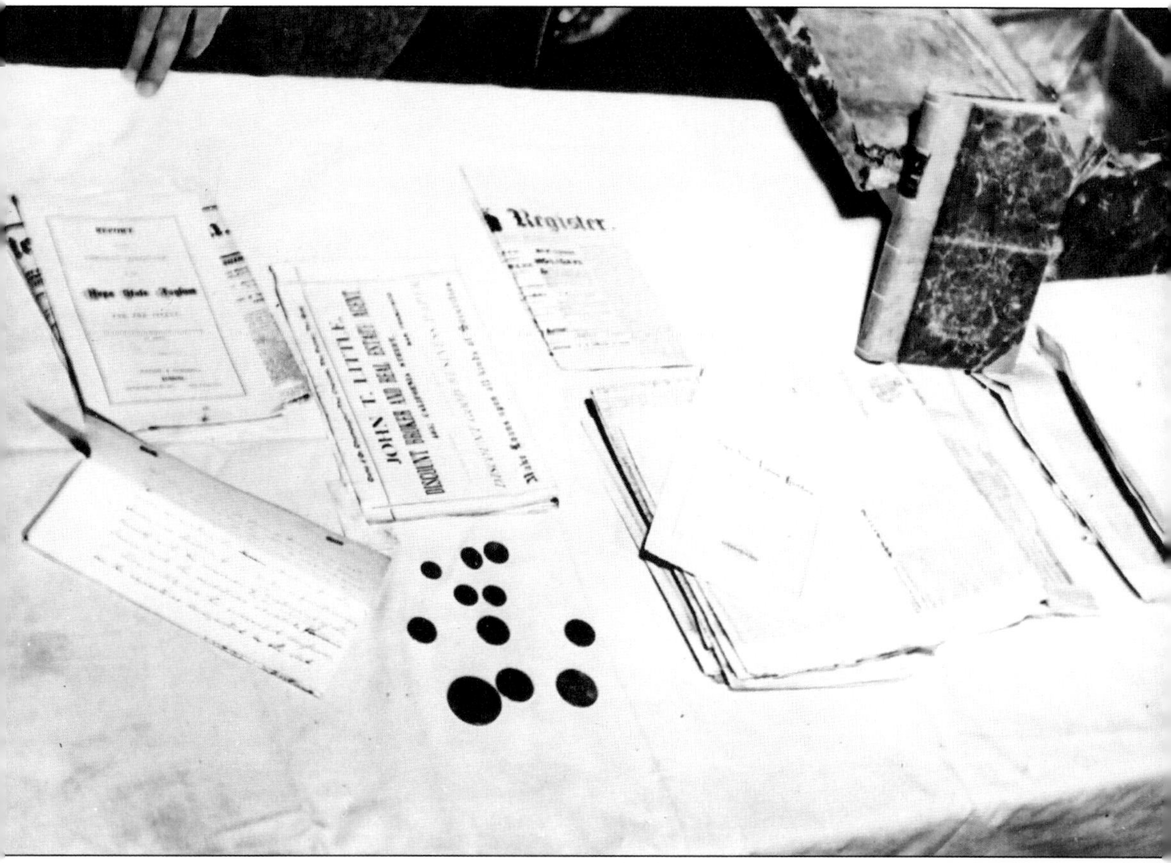

The copper cornerstone box, removed on June 22, 1949, contained the original Wright & Sanders blueprints for the hospital, a bound copy of Dr. Wilkins's survey report of 1871, a dedication report written by the board of directors, copies of the *Napa Register* and other California newspapers, reports on the Bank of Napa and Bank of Lake, a slip of paper autographed by a group of young witnesses, and several coins, including an Indian Head penny and a $2.50 gold coin. (Courtesy NCHS.)

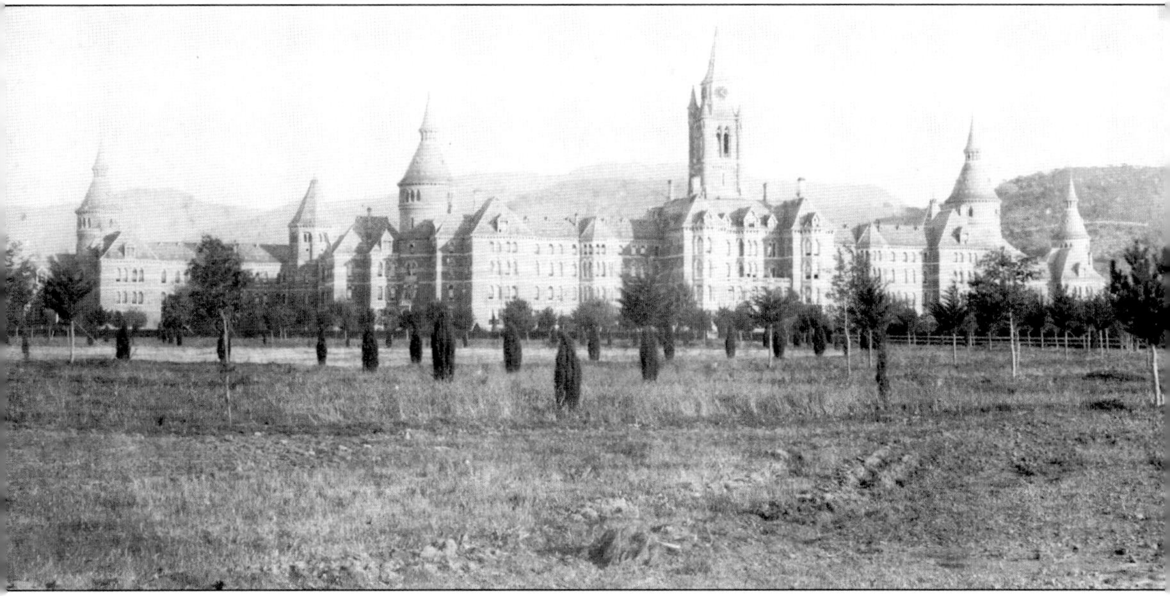

The Castle was completed for $1.5 million. The center wing was composed of the administrative department, visiting rooms, and officers' quarters. Directly above were residential apartments for the director on the second floor and the assistant physician on the third floor. Behind the first floor were a chapel and a library, along with separate service buildings for the main kitchen, bakery, laundry, and boiler room. Underneath the kitchen were three tunnels: one to the central section of the Castle and one to the last wings on either side of the Castle. Each tunnel had service pipes and cog railroad tracks for food and laundry carts. The two identical wings, which contained separate male and female wards, had single sleeping rooms, a dining room, and a central "living room" with an isinglass stove to evoke a tranquil setting. (Courtesy NCHS.)

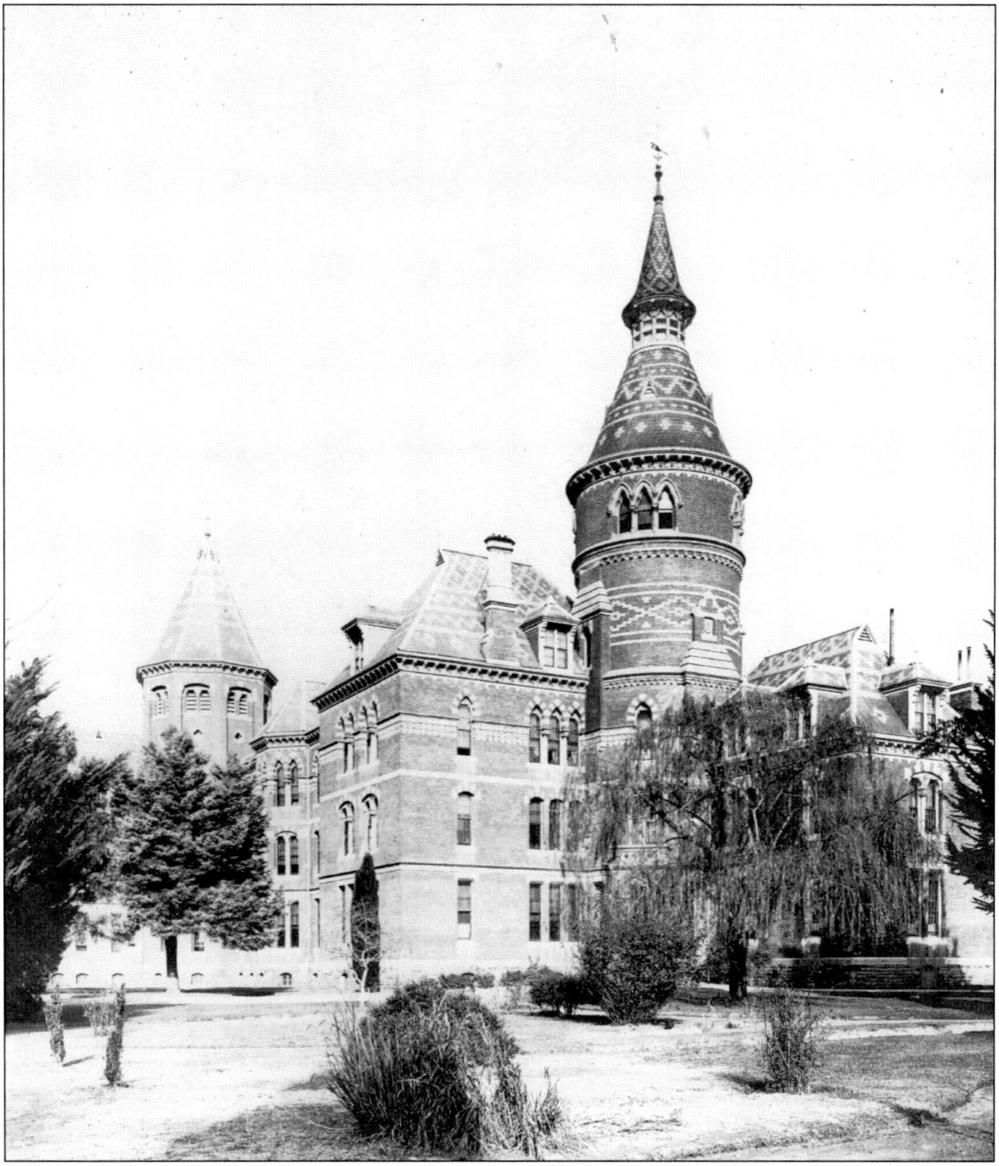

The imposing structure was forged of Vermont slate, Colfax marble with a Florentine-Moorish motif, and 10 million bricks, which were made in a factory set up on the site. There were seven towers with a $16,000 clock embedded in a central 175-foot tower. Shortly after 1906, the central tower was lowered to 60 feet due to damage from the San Francisco earthquake. The four round towers were used to store water for the gravity-flow elevator system, as well as for fire protection. The tower caps were removed after the 1906 earthquake and replaced with a flat roof to cover the water tanks. Precautions were taken as a result of the earthquake, when a patient building at Agnews State Hospital collapsed, killing 118 patients and staff. (Courtesy NCHS.)

The statues embedded in the entry arch represented the four basic cardinal virtues of ancient Greek philosophy: fortitude, justice, prudence, and temperance. The mottos over the forward-facing arches read: "In Temperance learn thou to live" (left); "Faith, hope and charity divine be thine beyond compare" (center); and "Let Prudence still thy footstep guide with Justice steadfast by her side" (right). (Courtesy NCHS.)

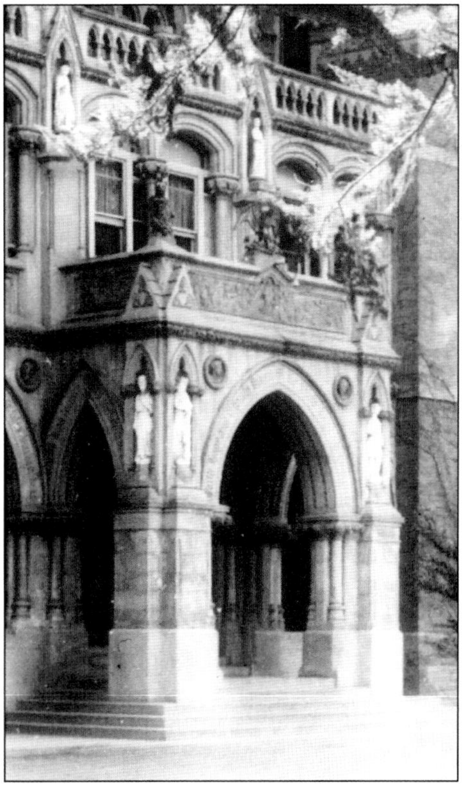

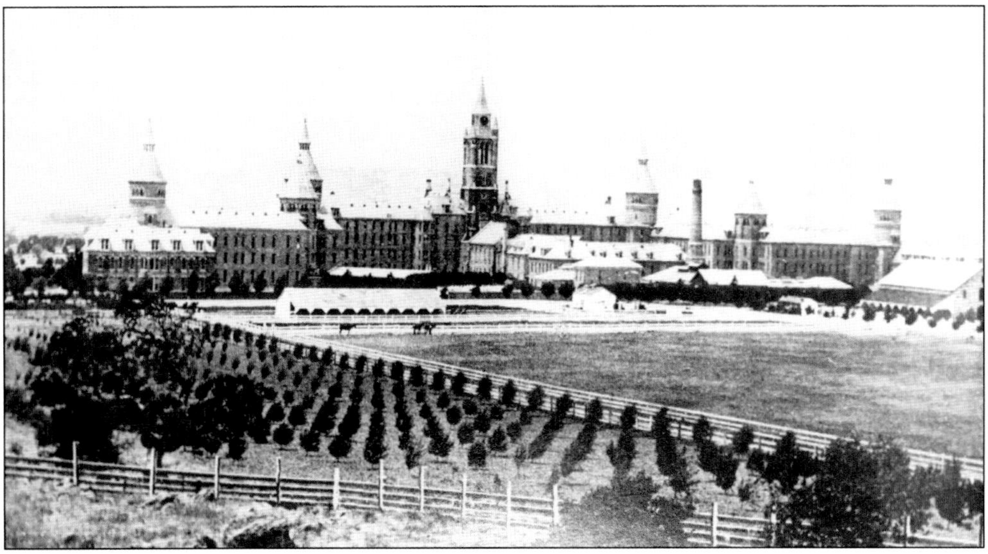

On April 19, 1876, a *San Francisco Chronicle* reporter remarked, "The ornate front entrance with its stone archways carved with quotations of possible biblical origin; the sculptured figures and other decorative carvings which surpasses the State Capitol, is more suitable for a home for millionaires than a housing place for the indigent insane." Political storms raged in Sacramento during the construction period. Democrats tried to sponsor a censure resolution charging "gross extravagance," while Republicans defended the expenditures. This view is of the rear orchards and the kitchen, laundry, and maintenance buildings. (Courtesy NSH.)

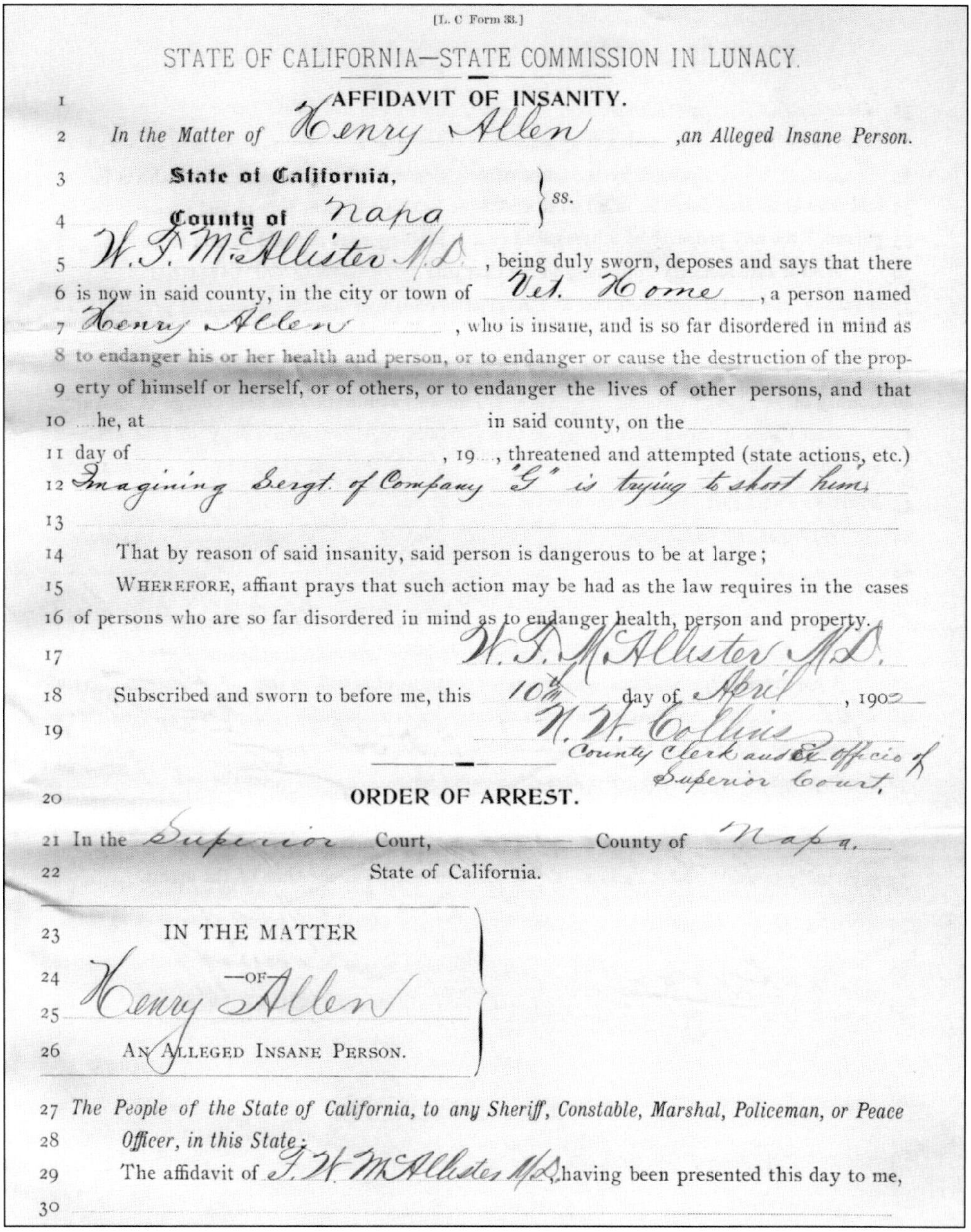

[L. C Form 33.]

STATE OF CALIFORNIA—STATE COMMISSION IN LUNACY.

AFFIDAVIT OF INSANITY.

In the Matter of Henry Allen *, an Alleged Insane Person.*

State of California, } ss.
County of Napa

W. F. McAllister M.D., being duly sworn, deposes and says that there is now in said county, in the city or town of Vet. Home, a person named Henry Allen, who is insane, and is so far disordered in mind as to endanger his or her health and person, or to endanger or cause the destruction of the property of himself or herself, or of others, or to endanger the lives of other persons, and that he, at in said county, on the day of , 19 , threatened and attempted (state actions, etc.) Imagining Sergt. of Company "G" is trying to shoot him.

That by reason of said insanity, said person is dangerous to be at large;

WHEREFORE, affiant prays that such action may be had as the law requires in the cases of persons who are so far disordered in mind as to endanger health, person and property.

W. F. McAllister M.D.

Subscribed and sworn to before me, this 10th day of April, 1902

N. W. Collins
County Clerk and Ex-Officio of Superior Court.

ORDER OF ARREST.

In the Superior Court, County of Napa.
State of California.

IN THE MATTER
—OF—
Henry Allen
AN ALLEGED INSANE PERSON.

The People of the State of California, to any Sheriff, Constable, Marshal, Policeman, or Peace Officer, in this State:

The affidavit of F. W. McAllister M.D. having been presented this day to me,

In this affidavit of insanity filed on April 10, 1902, a resident of the Yountville Veterans Home has been declared "insane, and [is] so far disordered in mind as to endanger his or her health and person . . . the destruction of the property . . . or to endanger the lives of other persons." The reason given is "imagining [the] Sergeant of Company 'G' is trying to shoot him." The majority of patients were committed by their families through the court system. A Complaint of Insanity was filed with the local magistrate, whereby a person was declared as "disordered of mind." A warrant was then issued, and the patient was taken into custody and examined by two doctors. Subsequently, he or she was formally committed during a hearing before the superior court judge. After the court hearing, the sheriff handcuffed the patient and then escorted him or her from the county courthouse to the Napa Asylum. (Courtesy NCHS.)

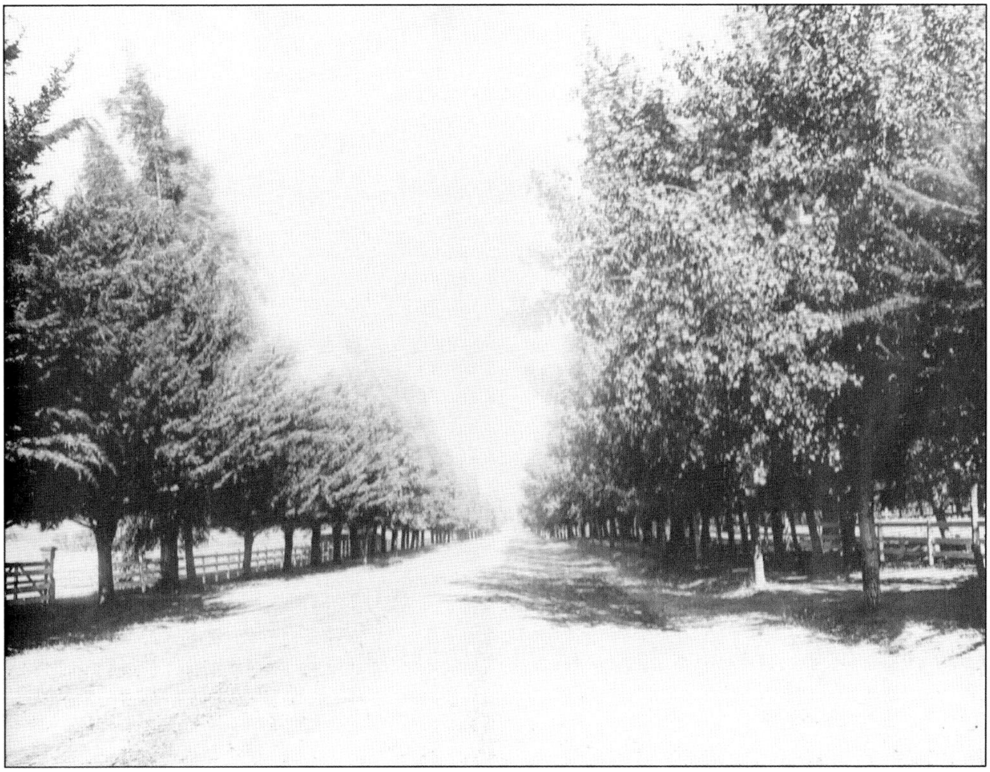

Magnolia Drive is seen here in a photograph taken from the front gate around 1890. To reach the hospital, visitors would travel by ferry, then walk, ride a horse, or take a wagon the three miles north to the hospital grounds. (Courtesy NSH.)

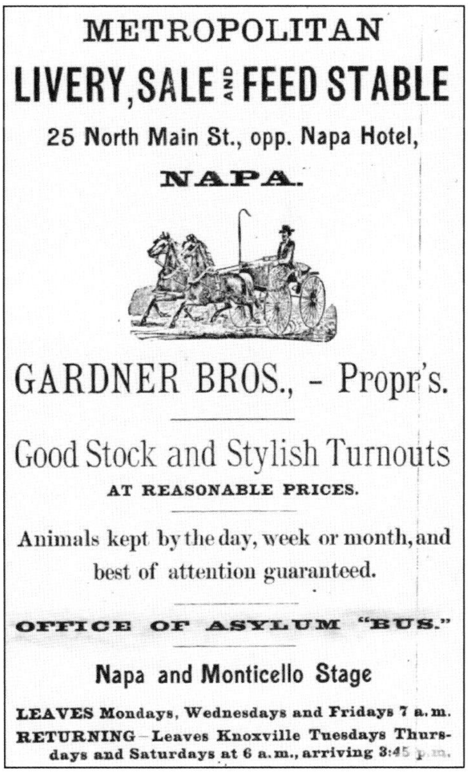

Travelers might have used a carriage from the Metropolitan Livery, Sale and Feed Stable, which offered up to five trips to the Napa Asylum, known locally as Imola. (Courtesy NCHS.)

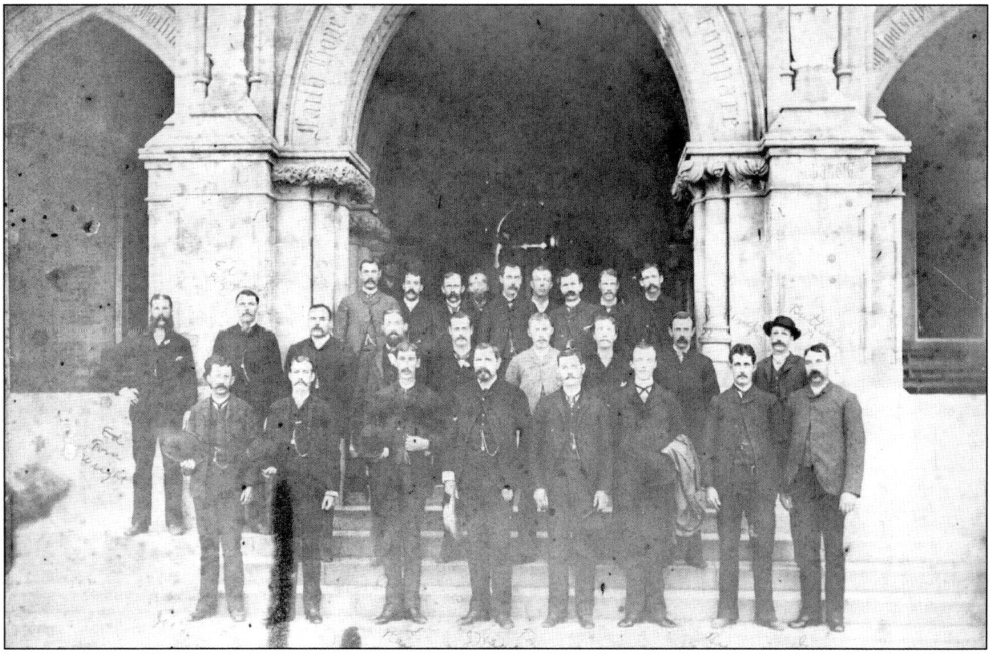

The staff was composed of 88 employees, including one resident physician, two assistant physicians, one secretary, one steward, one male and one female supervisor, one matron, one dispenser, four cooks, one secretary, one laundryman, three laundresses, one needlewoman, and 40 male and 30 female attendants. (Courtesy NCHS.)

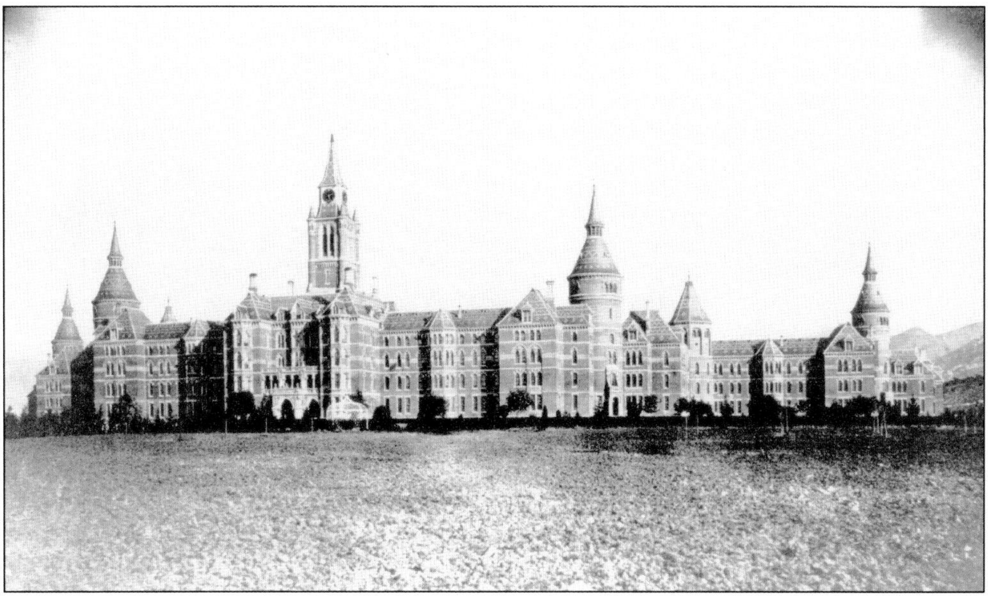

The first patient was admitted to the Napa Asylum for the Insane on November 15, 1875; in January 1876, the first patients were transferred from Stockton Asylum. Most of them were homeless or suffered from alcoholism. By 1880, the patient load had increased to such an extent that Superintendent Wilkins requested funds from the state to convert the attic areas into patient wards. In 1891, the asylum had 1,373 patients, which was double the amount it had been built to accommodate. (Courtesy Patricia Renait.)

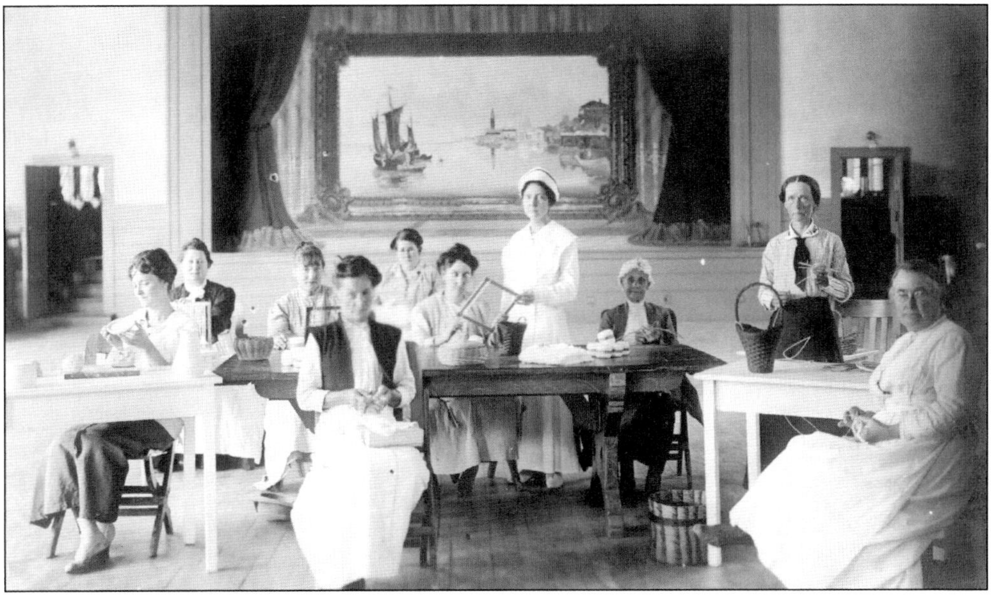

An early work therapy room in which patients are weaving baskets is pictured here about 1890. Maud Davis (center) was the supervising work therapy attendant. She was once commended for her "musical and elocutionary entertainments, given at various times to provide entertainment for the patients." (Courtesy NSH.)

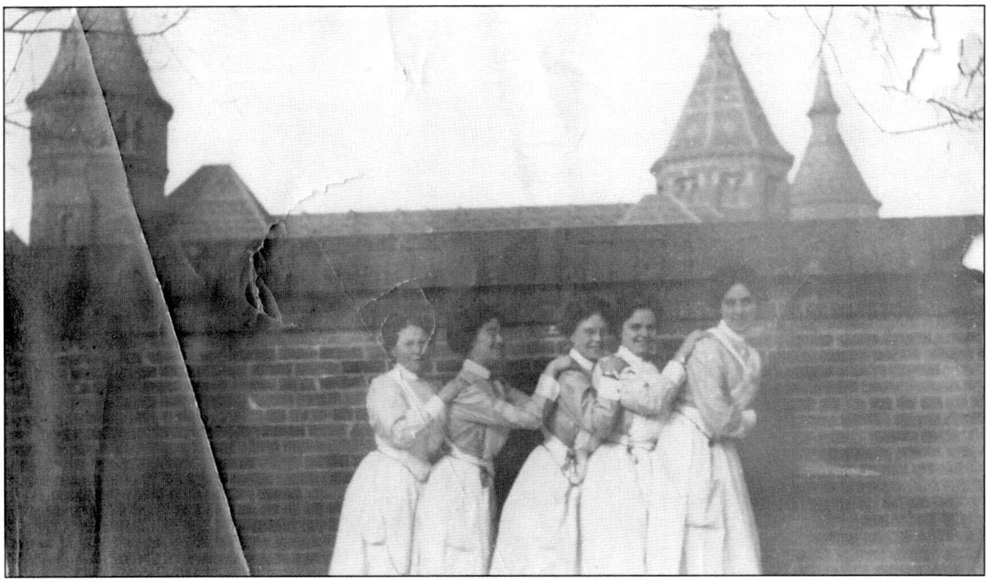

Staff lived on the same units as their patients, two to a room. Women who were drawn to asylum work were usually young, single, or widowed and "thrown upon their own resources." Asylum work offered an opportunity for women with limited education, knowledge of "domestic concerns," and a positive disposition. Young men who were not interested in farming or manual labor were also drawn to the relative security of working in an asylum. (Courtesy NCHS.)

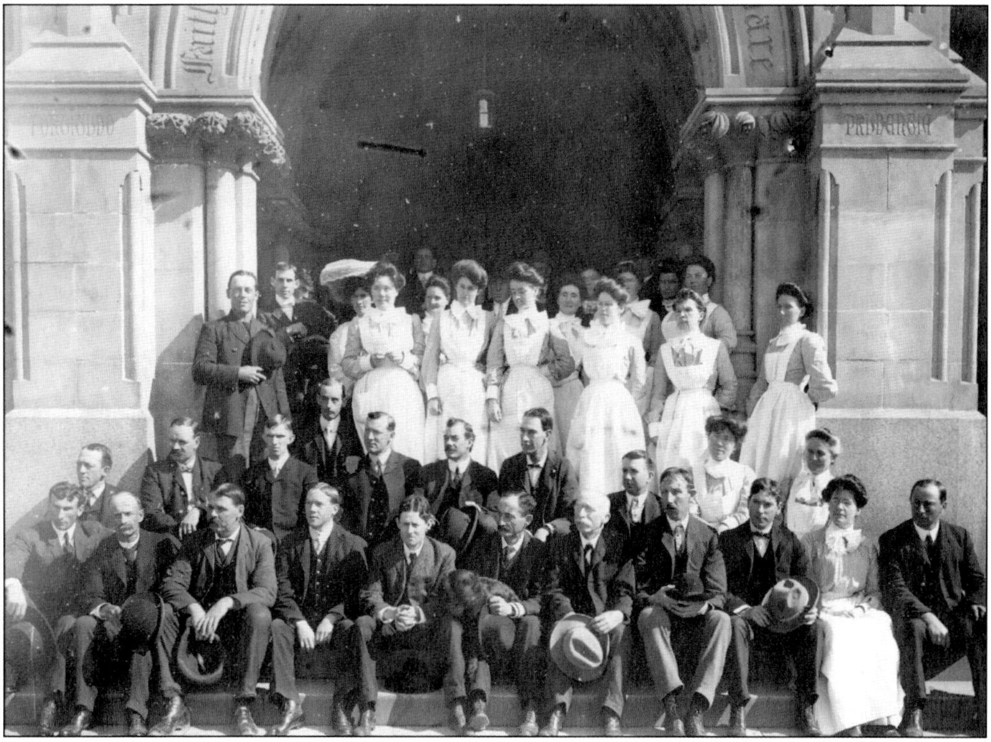

Ward attendants in 1900 earned a respectable living. Men earned $30 per month for the first six months, $35 the following year, and $40 "until promoted." Women in the same position earned $25 per month for the first six months, $30 the following year, and then $35 thereafter. The original working day started at 6:00 a.m. and ended at 9:00 p.m., with a half day off each week and one full day off per month. (Courtesy NSH.)

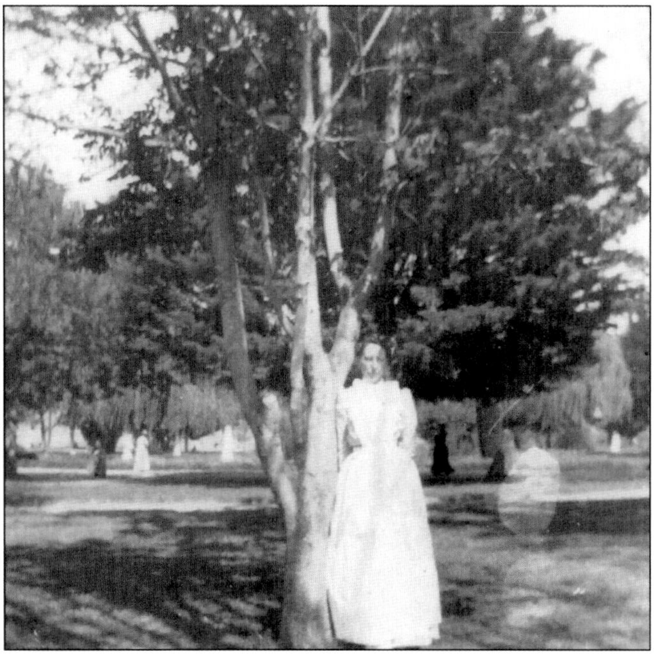

Mary Augusta "Molly" Williams Thompson, born in 1867, was a ward attendant who lived on the grounds with her youngest child, Robert. After becoming a widow at age 27, Molly had to earn a living to support her three children. She kept a small journal in which she made note of events: "Came to work at asylum April 3, 1895," and "Big earthquake April 18, 1906." In 1922, Molly married Alonzo J. Vanderhoff, a widower who also worked at the asylum. (Courtesy Patricia Renait.)

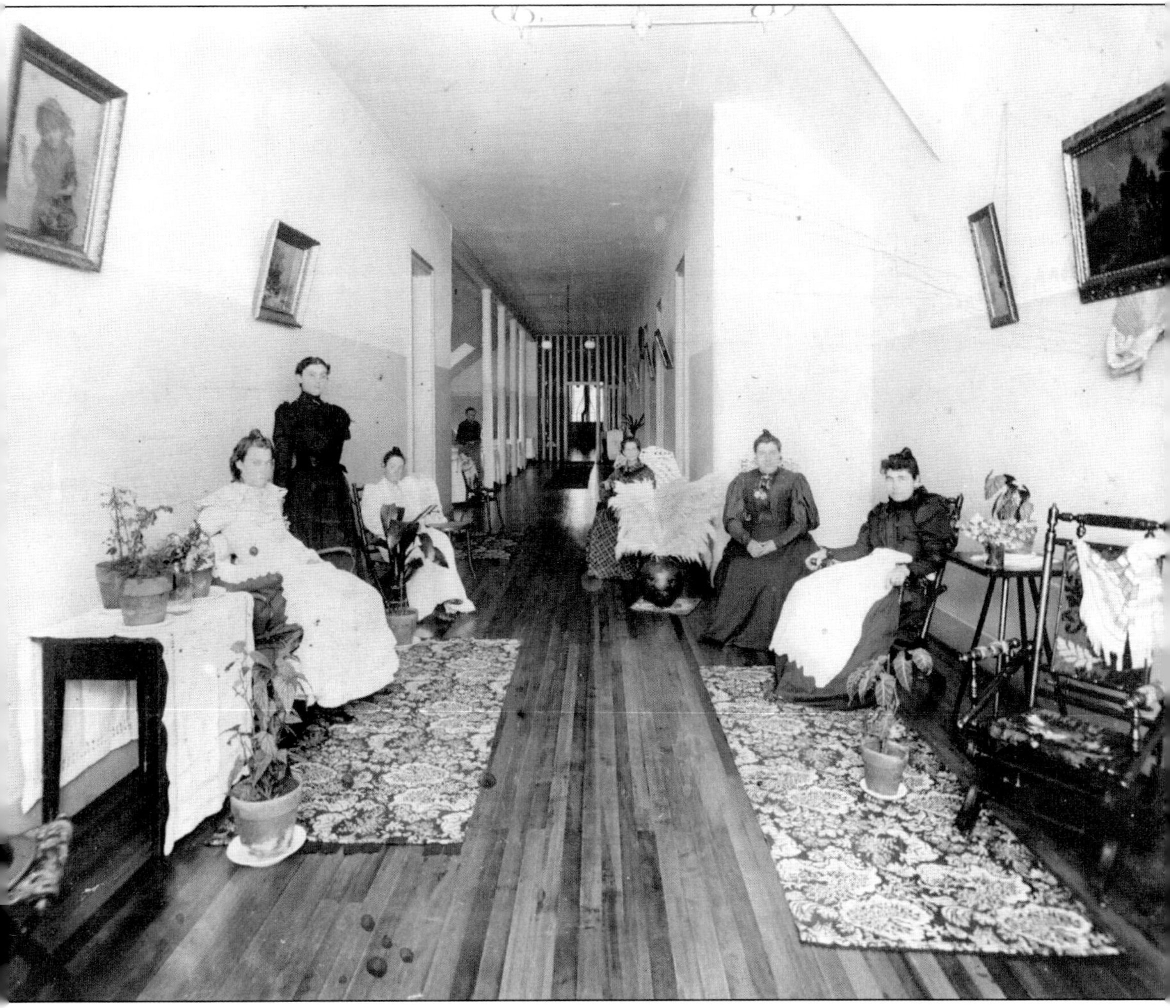

In this unidentified living room of a women's ward around 1890, the ward matron, wearing black, is seen standing on the left. The quiet, more socially acceptable patients were given grounds privileges and were housed in the units closest to the central section. Violent and unmanageable patients were housed in separate rooms on the ends of the wings. These rooms contained very few furnishings in order to prevent injuries to themselves or others. (Courtesy NCHS.)

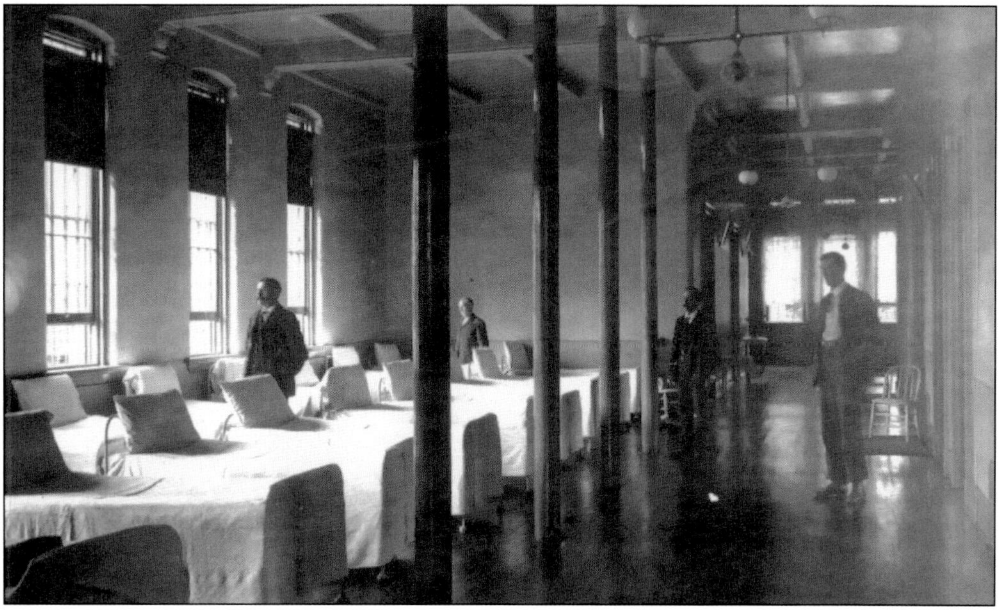

Pictured here is one of the attic wards at the turn of the 20th century. The regular wards had one dormitory area for six beds, one 10-foot-by-10-foot room for two beds, and thirteen 8-foot-by-10-foot rooms with one bed each in addition to an attendant's room, dining room, pantry, clothes room, bathroom, washroom, and closets. Each room had large windows with security bars on the exterior. (Courtesy NSH.)

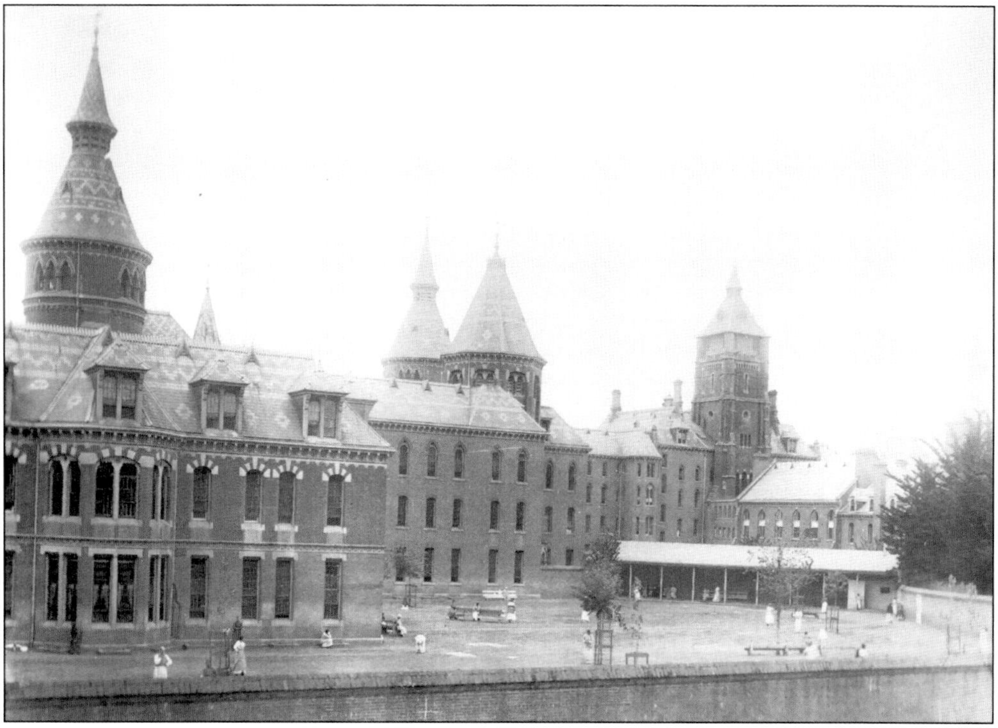

In 1898, the majority of women were diagnosed with acute mania, melancholia, or paranoia. Here is one of the few images of the south wing and female yard. (Courtesy CSA.)

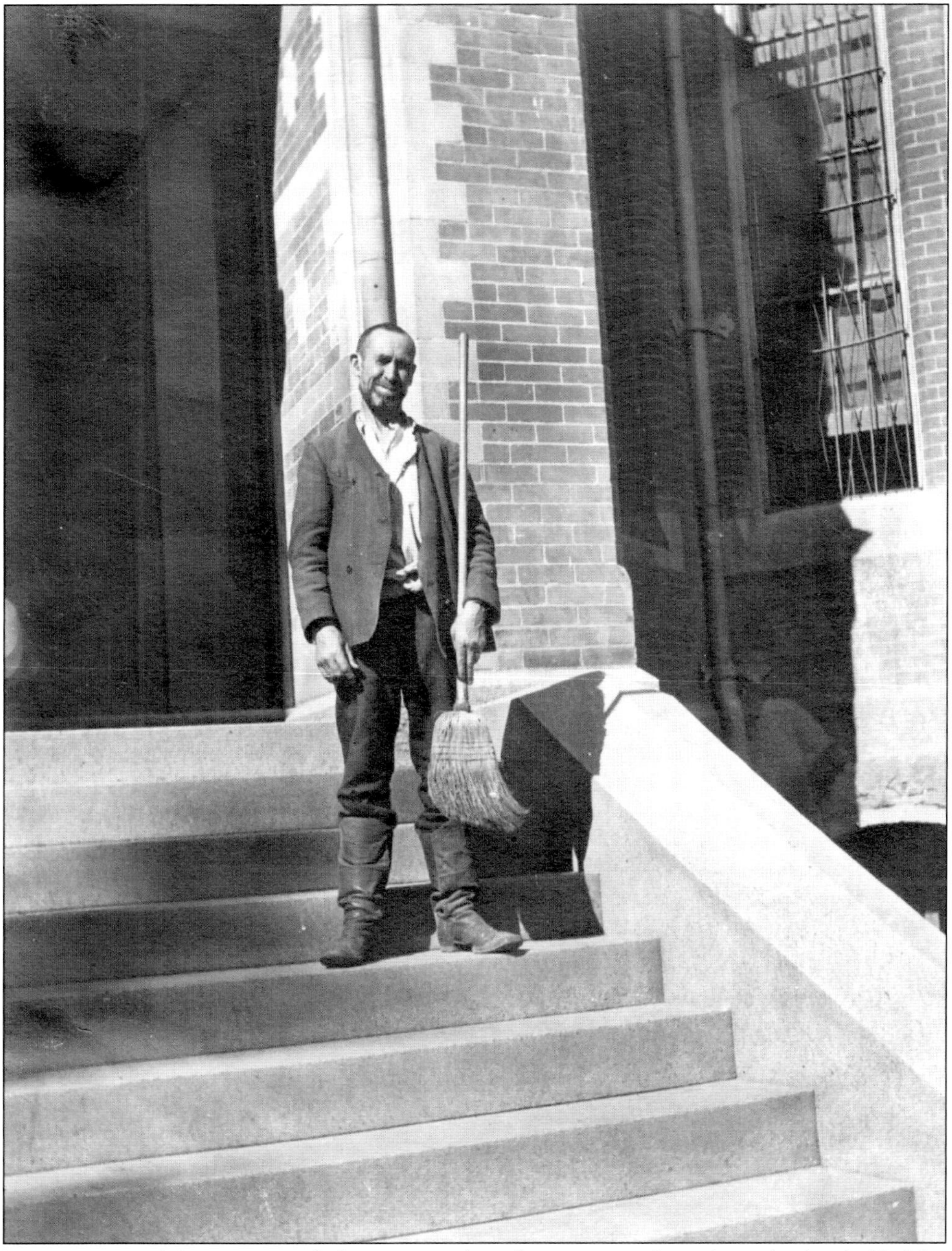

Men constituted the majority of admissions and resident patients throughout the first half of the 20th century. (Courtesy NSH.)

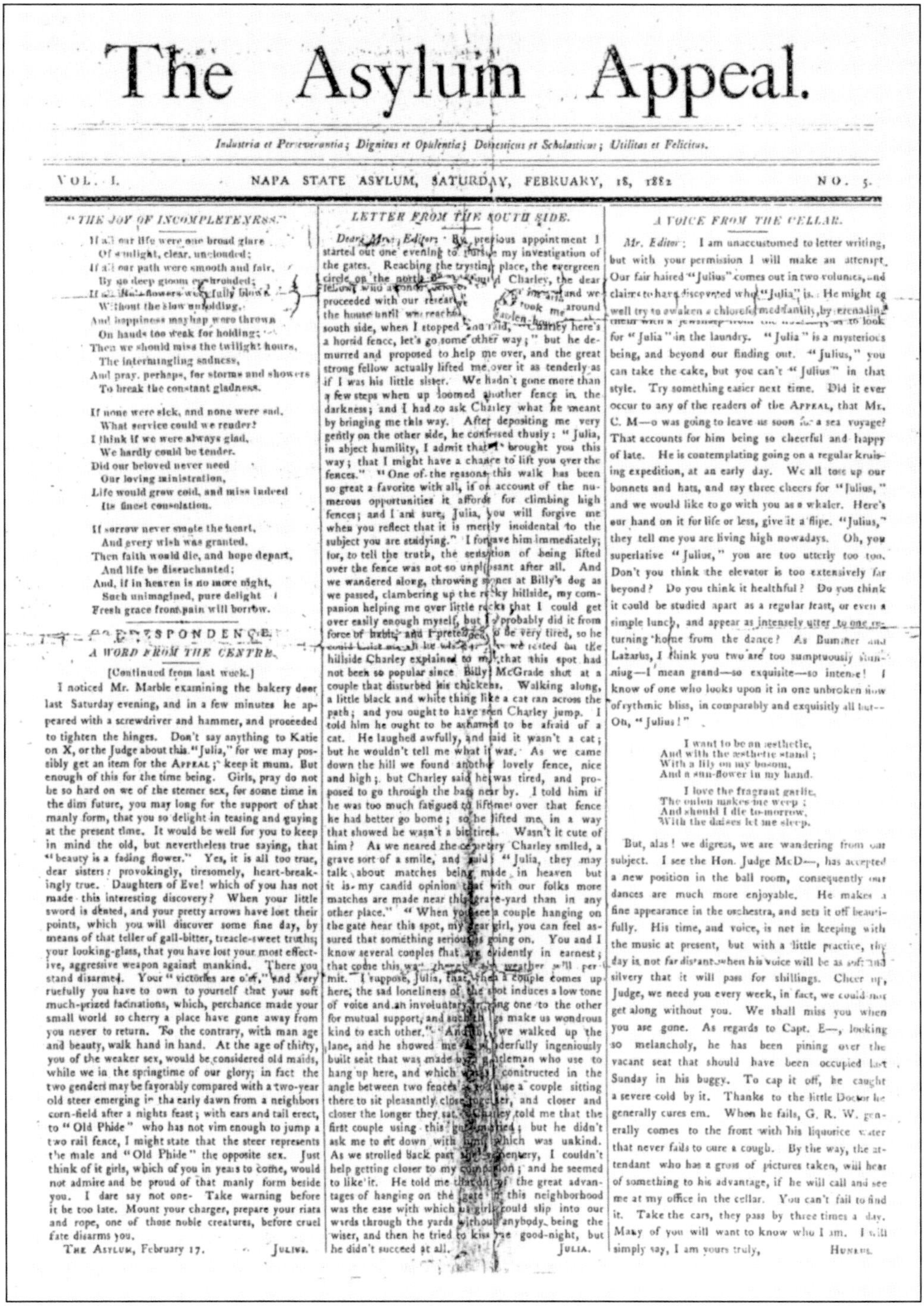

The Asylum Appeal.

Industria et Perseverantia; Dignitas et Opulentia; Domesticus et Scholasticus; Utilitas et Felicitas.

VOL. I. NAPA STATE ASYLUM, SATURDAY, FEBRUARY, 18, 1882 NO. 5.

"THE JOY OF INCOMPLETENESS."

If all our life were one broad glare
Of sunlight, clear, unclouded;
If all our path were smooth and fair,
By no deep gloom enshrouded;
If all life's flowers were fully blown
Without the slow unfolding,
And happiness mayhap were thrown
On hands too weak for holding;
Then we should miss the twilight hours,
The intermingling sadness,
And pray, perhaps, for storms and showers
To break the constant gladness.

If none were sick, and none were sad,
What service could we render?
I think if we were always glad,
We hardly could be tender.
Did our beloved never need
Our loving ministration,
Life would grow cold, and miss indeed
Its finest consolation.

If sorrow never smote the heart,
And every wish was granted,
Then faith would die, and hope depart,
And life be disenchanted;
And, if in heaven is no more night,
Such unimagined, pure delight
Fresh grace from pain will borrow.

CORRESPONDENCE.

A WORD FROM THE CENTRE.

[Continued from last week.]

I noticed Mr. Marble examining the bakery door last Saturday evening, and in a few minutes he appeared with a screwdriver and hammer, and proceeded to tighten the hinges. Don't say anything to Katie on X, or the Judge about this "Julia," for we may possibly get an item for the APPEAL; keep it mum. But enough of this for the time being. Girls, pray do not be so hard on we of the sterner sex, for some time in the dim future, you may long for the support of that manly form, that you so delight in teasing and guying at the present time. It would be well for you to keep in mind the old, but nevertheless true saying, that "beauty is a fading flower." Yes, it is all too true, dear sisters: provokingly, tiresomely, heart-breakingly true. Daughters of Eve! which of you has not made this interesting discovery? When your little sword is dented, and your pretty arrows have lost their points, which you will discover some fine day, by means of that teller of gall-bitter, treacle-sweet truths; your looking-glass, that you have lost your most effective, aggressive weapon against mankind. There you stand disarmed. Your "victories are o'ef," and very ruefully you have to own to yourself that your soft much-prized facinations, which, perchance made your small world so cherry a place have gone away from you never to return. To the contrary, with man age and beauty, walk hand in hand. At the age of thirty, you of the weaker sex, would be considered old maids, while we in the springtime of our glory; in fact the two genders may be fayorably compared with a two-year old steer emerging in tha early dawn from a neighbors corn-field after a nights feast; with ears and tail erect, to "Old Phide" who has not vim enough to jump a two rail fence, I might state that the steer represents the male and "Old Phide" the opposite sex. Just think of it girls, which of you in years to come, would not admire and be proud of that manly form beside you. I dare say not one. Take warning before it be too late. Mount your charger, prepare your riata and rope, one of those noble creatures, before cruel fate disarms you.

THE ASYLUM, February 17. JULIUS.

LETTER FROM THE SOUTH SIDE.

Dear Mr. Editor: By previous appointment I started out one evening to pursue my investigation of the gates. Reaching the trysting place, the evergreen circle on the north [illegible] Charley, the dear fellow who [illegible] and we proceeded with our research [illegible] took me around the house until we reached [illegible] garden-house [illegible] south side, when I stopped and said, "Charley here's a horrid fence, let's go some other way;" but he demurred and proposed to help me over, and the great strong fellow actually lifted me over it as tenderly as if I was his little sister. We hadn't gone more than a few steps when up loomed another fence in the darkness; and I had to ask Charley what he meant by bringing me this way. After depositing me very gently on the other side, he confessed thusly: "Julia, in abject humility, I admit that I brought you this way; that I might have a chance to lift you over the fences." "One of the reasons this walk has been so great a favorite with all, is on account of the numerous opportunities it affords for climbing high fences; and I am sure, Julia, you will forgive me when you reflect that it is merely incidental to the subject you are studying." I forgave him immediately; for, to tell the truth, the sensation of being lifted over the fence was not so unpleasant after all. And we wandered along, throwing stones at Billy's dog as we passed, clambering up the rocky hillside, my companion helping me over little rocks that I could get over easily enough myself, but I probably did it from force of habit, and I pretended to be very tired, so he could [illegible] we rested on the hillside Charley explained to me that this spot had not been so popular since Billy McGrade shot at a couple that disturbed his chickens. Walking along, a little black and white thing like a cat ran across the path; and you ought to have seen Charley jump. I told him he ought to be ashamed to be afraid of a cat. He laughed awfully, and said it wasn't a cat; but he wouldn't tell me what it was. As we came down the hill we found another lovely fence, nice and high; but Charley said he was tired, and proposed to go through the bars near by. I told him if he was too much fatigued to lift me over that fence he had better go home; so he lifted me in a way that showed he wasn't a bit tired. Wasn't it cute of him? As we neared the cemetery Charley smiled, a grave sort of a smile, and said: "Julia, they may talk about matches being made in heaven but it is my candid opinion that with our folks more matches are made near this grave-yard than in any other place." "When you see a couple hanging on the gate near this spot, my dear girl, you can feel assured that something serious is going on. You and I know several couples that are evidently in earnest; that come this way [illegible] weather will permit. I suppose, Julia, that when a couple comes up here, the sad loneliness of the spot induces a low tone of voice and an involuntary [illegible] one to the other for mutual support, and such things make us wondrous kind to each other." And [illegible] we walked up the lane, and he showed me a wonderfully ingeniously built seat that was made by a gentleman who use to hang up here, and which [illegible] constructed in the angle between two fences [illegible] a couple sitting there to sit pleasantly close together, and closer and closer the longer they sat. Charley told me that the first couple using this [illegible] married; but he didn't ask me to sit down with him, which was unkind. As we strolled back past the cemetery, I couldn't help getting closer to my companion; and he seemed to like it. He told me that one of the great advantages of hanging on the gate in this neighborhood was the ease with which us girls could slip into our wards through the yards without anybody being the wiser, and then he tried to kiss me good-night, but he didn't succeed at all. JULIA.

A VOICE FROM THE CELLAR.

Mr. Editor: I am unaccustomed to letter writing, but with your permission I will make an attempt. Our fair haired "Julius" comes out in two volumes, and claims to have discovered who "Julia" is. He might as well try to awaken a chloroformed family by serenading them with a [illegible] to look for "Julia" in the laundry. "Julia" is a mysterious being, and beyond our finding out. "Julius," you can take the cake, but you can't "Julius" in that style. Try something easier next time. Did it ever occur to any of the readers of the APPEAL, that Mr. C. M—o was going to leave us soon for a sea voyage? That accounts for him being so cheerful and happy of late. He is contemplating going on a regular kruising expedition, at an early day. We all toss up our bonnets and hats, and say three cheers for "Julius," and we would like to go with you as a whaler. Here's our hand on it for life or less, give it a flipe. "Julius," they tell me you are living high nowadays. Oh, you superlative "Julius," you are too utterly too too. Don't you think the elevator is too extensively far beyond? Do you think it healthful? Do you think it could be studied apart as a regular feast, or even a simple lunch, and appear as intensely utter to one returning home from the dance? As Bummer and Lazarus, I think you two are too sumptuously stunning—I mean grand—so exquisite—so intense! I know of one who looks upon it in one unbroken flow of rythmic bliss, in comparably and exquisitly all but— Oh, "Julius!"

I want to be an æsthetic,
And with the æsthetic stand;
With a lily on my bosom,
And a sun-flower in my hand.

I love the fragrant garlic,
The onion makes me weep;
And should I die to-morrow,
With the daises let me sleep.

But, alas! we digress, we are wandering from our subject. I see the Hon. Judge McD—, has accepted a new position in the ball room, consequently our dances are much more enjoyable. He makes a fine appearance in the orchestra, and sets it off beautifully. His time, and voice, is not in keeping with the music at present, but with a little practice, the day is not far distant when his voice will be as soft and silvery that it will pass for shillings. Cheer up, Judge, we need you every week, in fact, we could not get along without you. We shall miss you when you are gone. As regards to Capt. E—, looking so melancholy, he has been pining over the vacant seat that should have been occupied last Sunday in his buggy. To cap it off, he caught a severe cold by it. Thanks to the little Doctor he generally cures em. When he fails, G. R. W. generally comes to the front with his liquorice water that never fails to cure a cough. By the way, the attendant who has a gross of pictures taken, will hear of something to his advantage, if he will call and see me at my office in the cellar. You can't fail to find it. Take the cars, they pass by three times a day. Many of you will want to know who I am. I will simply say, I am yours truly, HUNKUS.

The *Asylum Appeal* was written and printed by John Donovan, a patient. It provided "more reading matter for the patients than ever before known." The newsletter included poetry, letters from patients to the editor, articles on the goings-on of the asylum, various observances and jokes, weather reports, and local advertisements. Donovan reportedly disappeared into the hills and returned after some months. (Courtesy NCHS.)

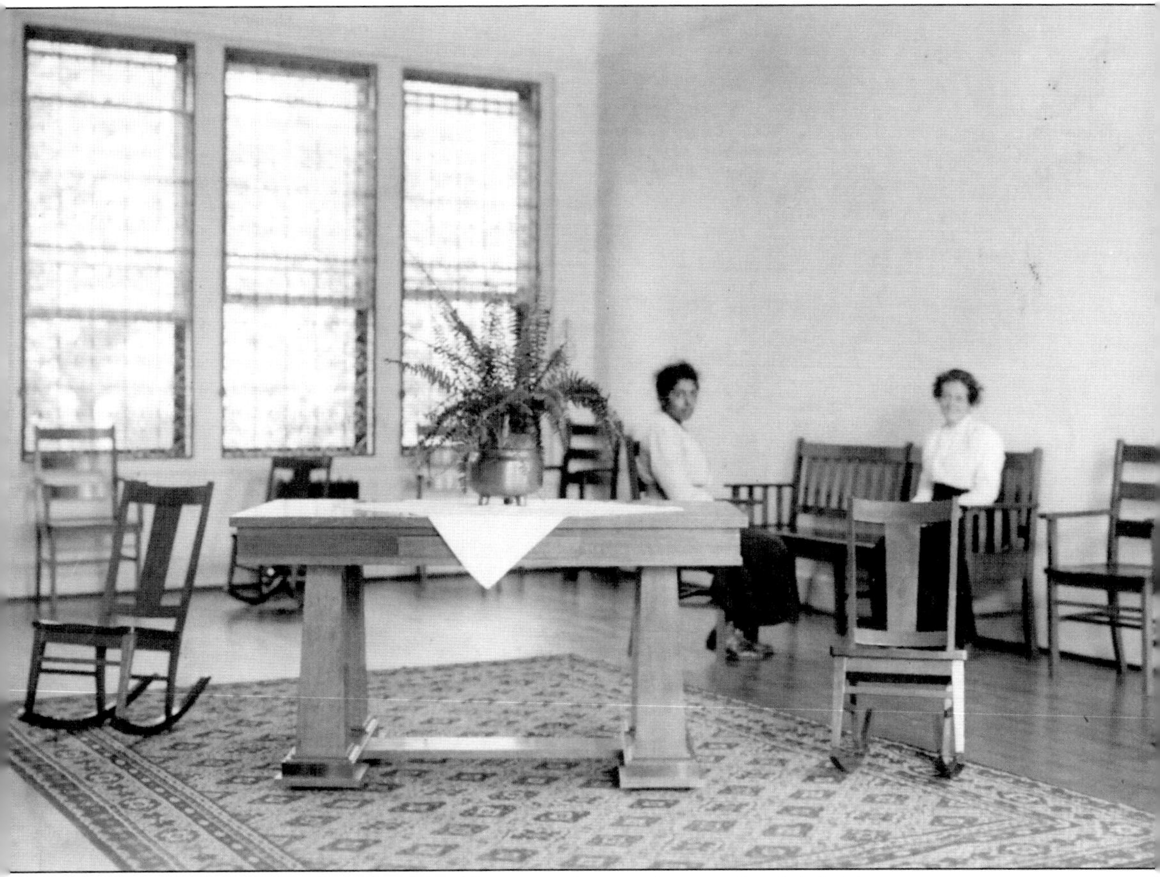

Most patients were admitted from San Francisco County, but another 26 California counties were represented as well. In this era, among the stated reasons for admission were business troubles, childbirth, use of opium, typhoid fever, sunstroke, spiritualism, paralysis, overwork, jealousy, heredity, grief, epilepsy, domestic trouble, disappointment in love, loss in mining stocks, masturbation, sensational reading, syphilis, and excessive study. The asylum intended to provide a homelike setting for convalescence as illustrated with this sitting room. (Courtesy NCHS.)

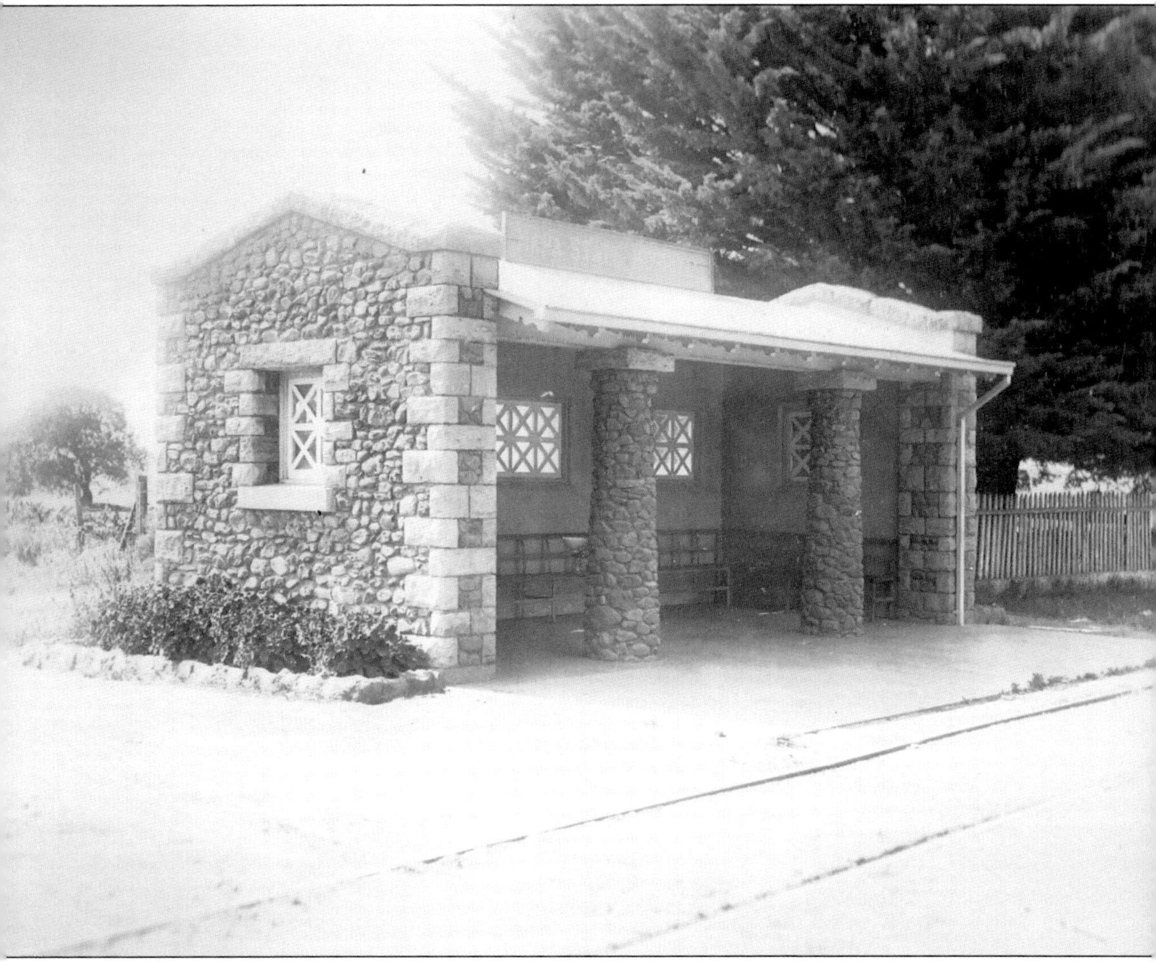

The bus shelter, built in 1910, was the waiting area for passengers riding the San Francisco, Napa & Calistoga Railway. The electric line, which started in 1905, ran six times a day from Vallejo to Napa by 1912. (Courtesy CSA.)

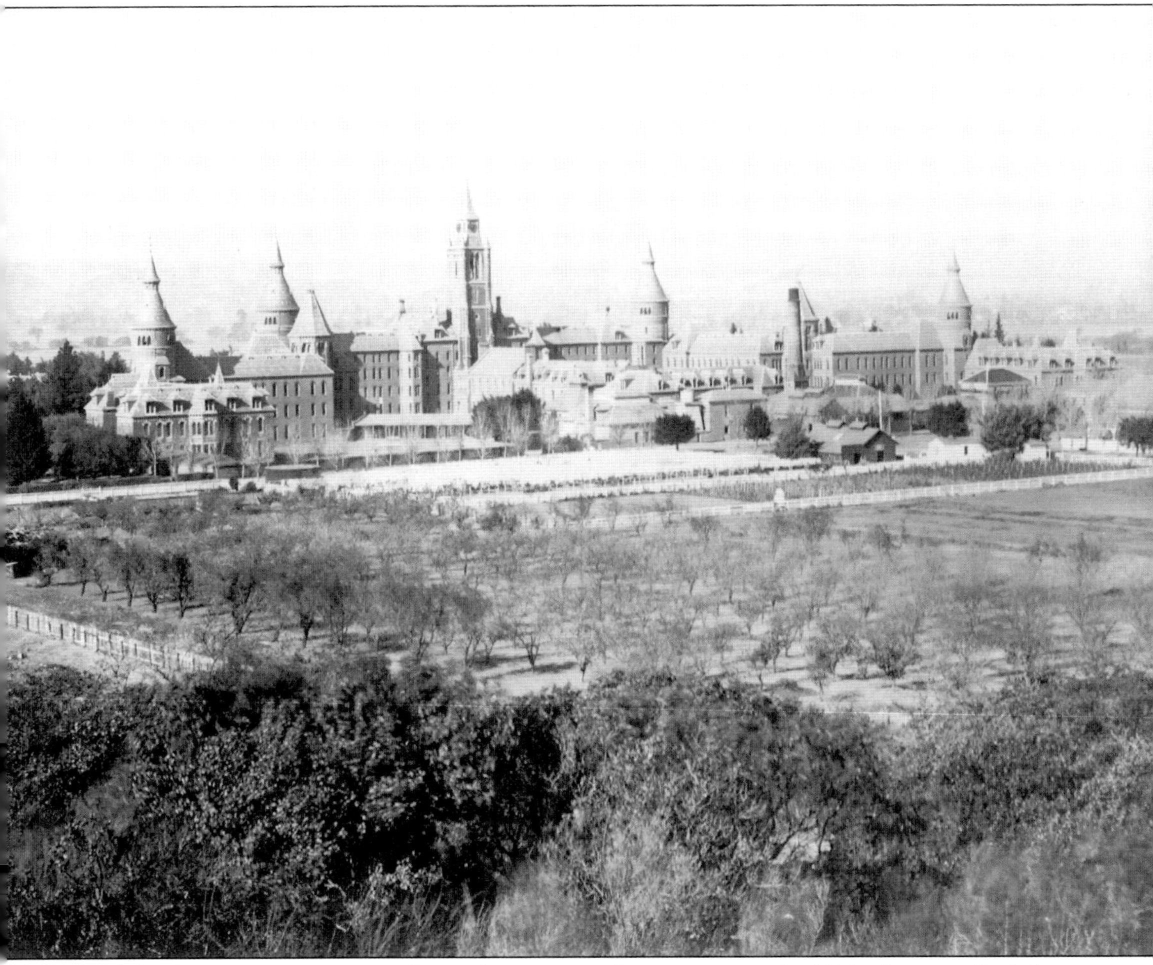

Imola had a major economic and social impact on the community. In 1901, the payroll of the asylum's 200 employees was more than Napa County's entire state tax bill. In order to provide mail services to an increasing number of patients and staff, a US government post office was established on September 21, 1921. It was called the Imola Post Office, and mail sent to the asylum was addressed to Imola, California. (Courtesy NCHS.)

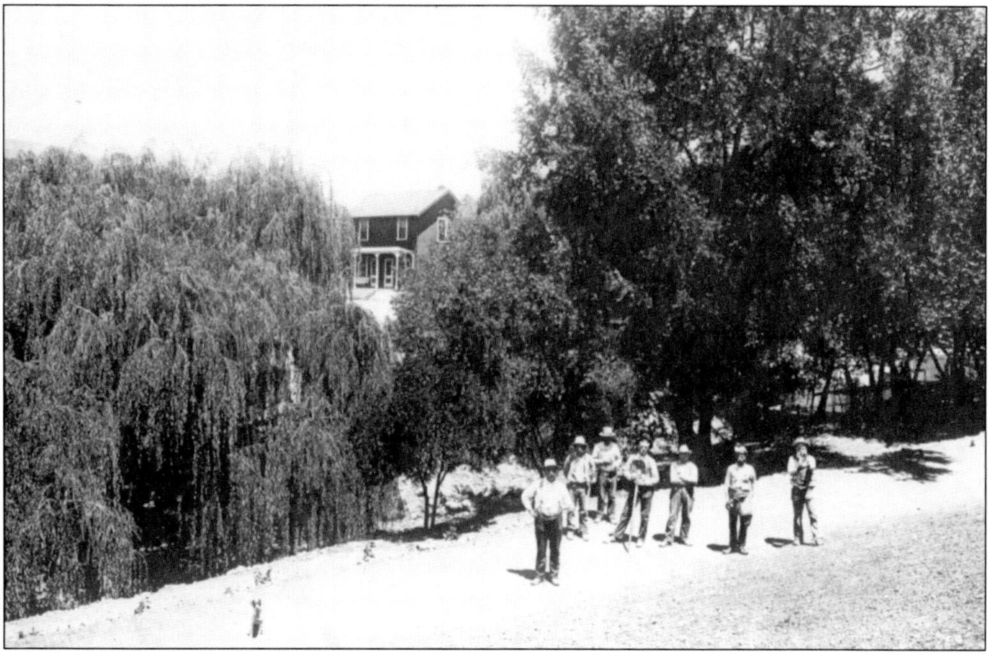

Guided by the principles of moral treatment, the hospital promoted the health benefits of farm labor. The 1882 annual report stated that the per capita expense of 42¢ per day would not be possible without the "products of the farm, garden, and dairy, which were the fruits of labor mostly done by the patients." (Courtesy CSA.)

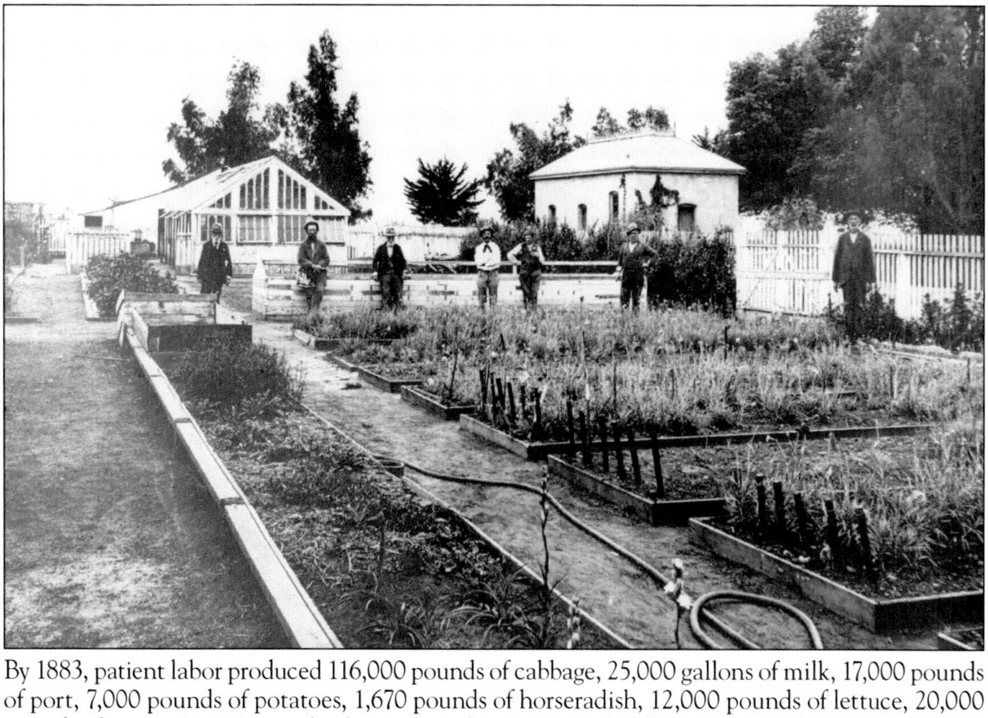

By 1883, patient labor produced 116,000 pounds of cabbage, 25,000 gallons of milk, 17,000 pounds of port, 7,000 pounds of potatoes, 1,670 pounds of horseradish, 12,000 pounds of lettuce, 20,000 pounds of grapes, 33,000 pounds of turnips, and 18,000 pounds of beets. Surplus fruit and vegetables were canned on-site and sent out to other state hospitals. (Courtesy NSH.)

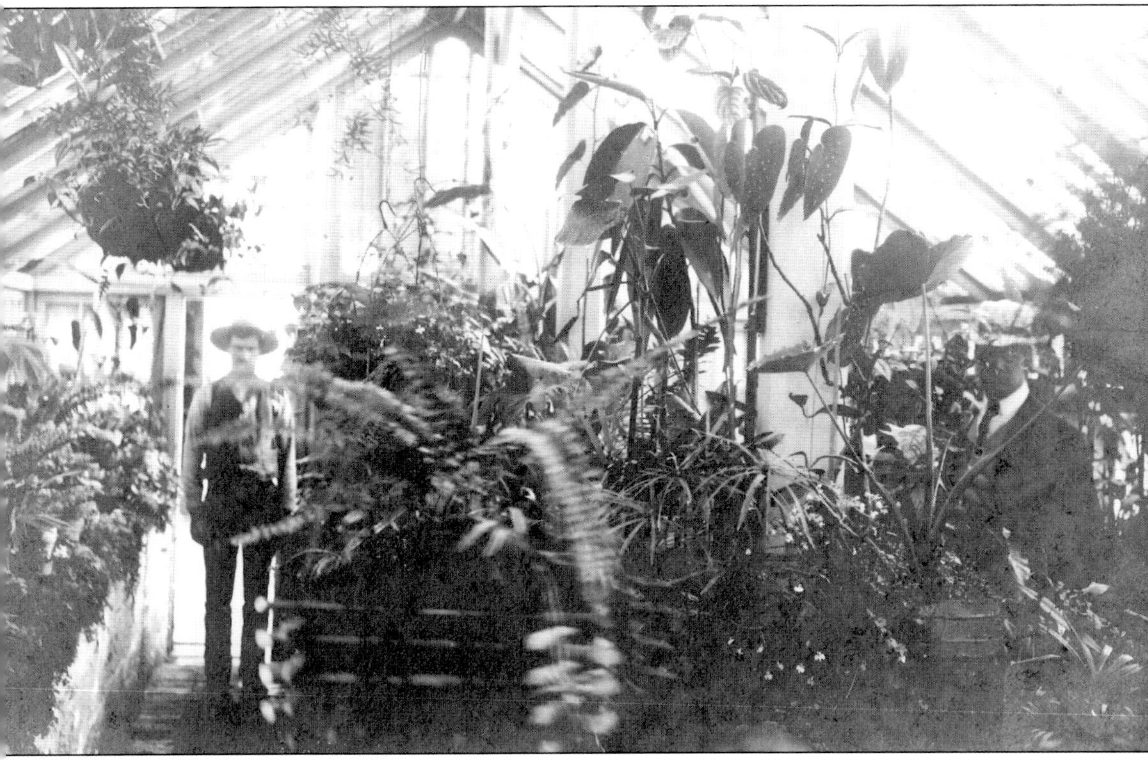

Flowers from the arboretum were used to brighten up hospital wards and to teach patients the art of flower arranging. An average of 40 to 50 patients were assigned to the nursery and other landscaped areas for work therapy. Tom Donohue, the groundskeeper, is pictured here around the turn of the 20th century. (Courtesy NCHS.)

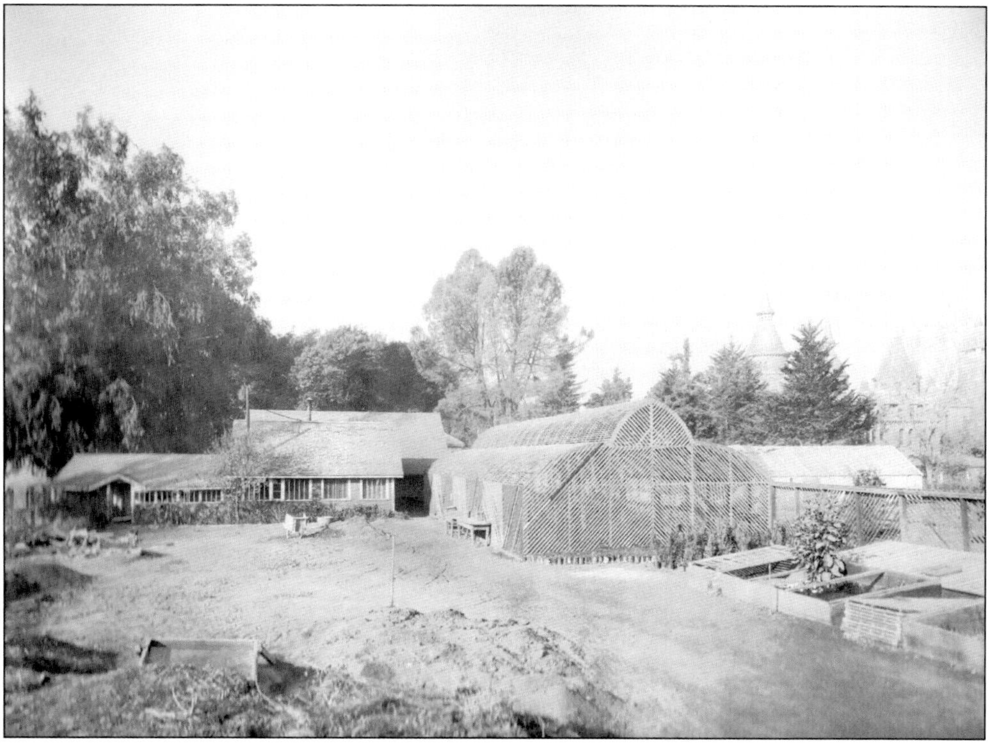

In this rear view of the greenhouses, the Castle towers are visible in the distance. The hothouses were partially constructed of bricks made at the on-site factory. (Courtesy CSA.)

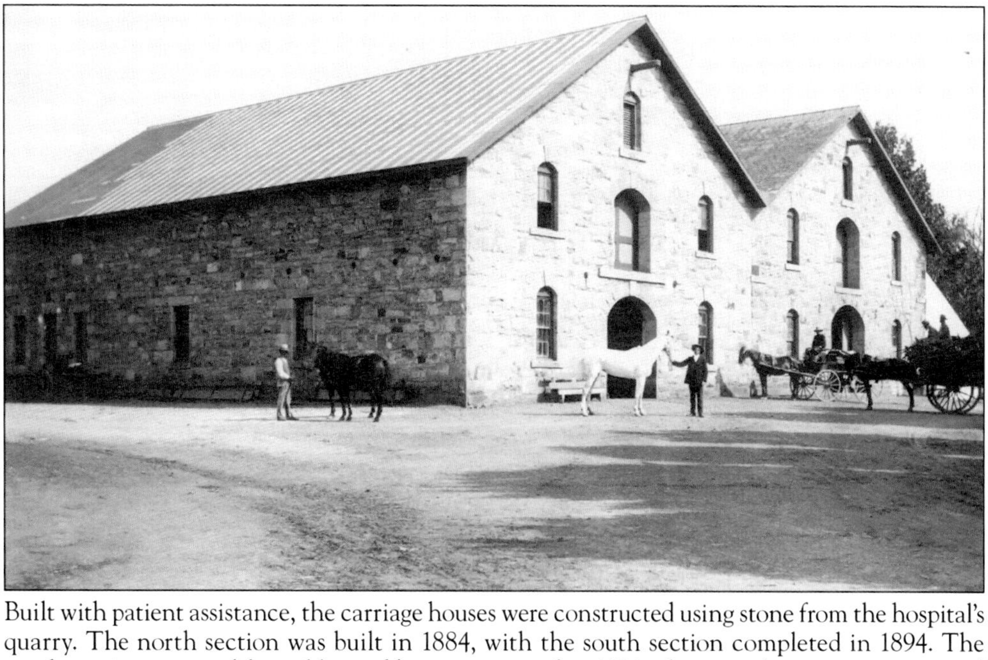

Built with patient assistance, the carriage houses were constructed using stone from the hospital's quarry. The north section was built in 1884, with the south section completed in 1894. The north section was used for stables and hay storage, and in 1914 it became the carpentry, tin, and upholstery shops. The entire lower level later became the Dolly Shop, and a Pallid Bat Colony moved in upstairs. (Courtesy NSH.)

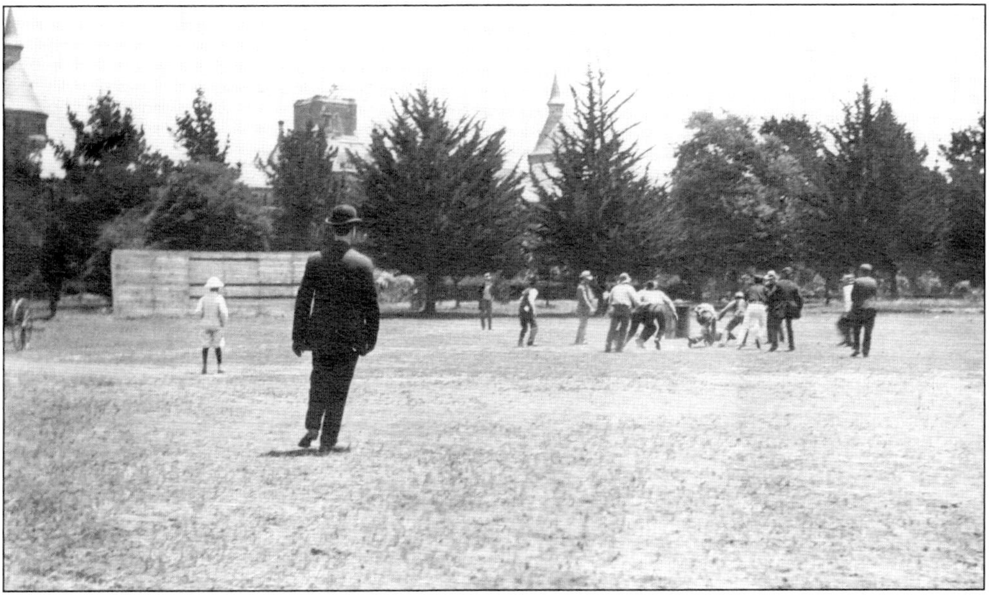

Pictured here around 1905, the baseball diamond provided a much-needed physical outlet for patients and community members. (Courtesy NSH.)

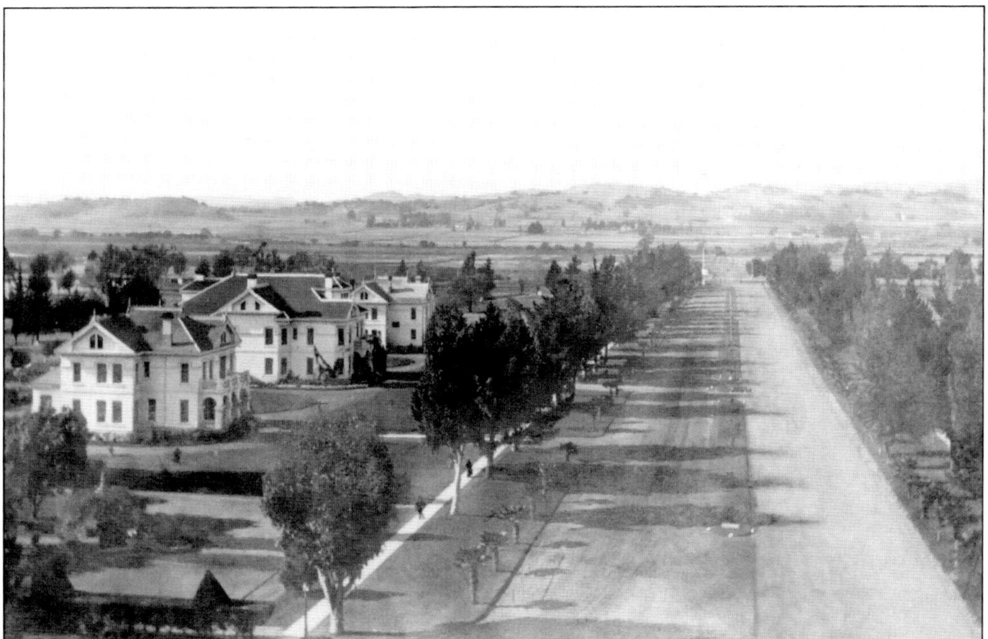

Dr. Wilkins had to request money from the state several times before $12,000 was allocated for these residence "cottages." Once built, the doctor's quarters in the Castle were converted to patient wards. (Courtesy NSH.)

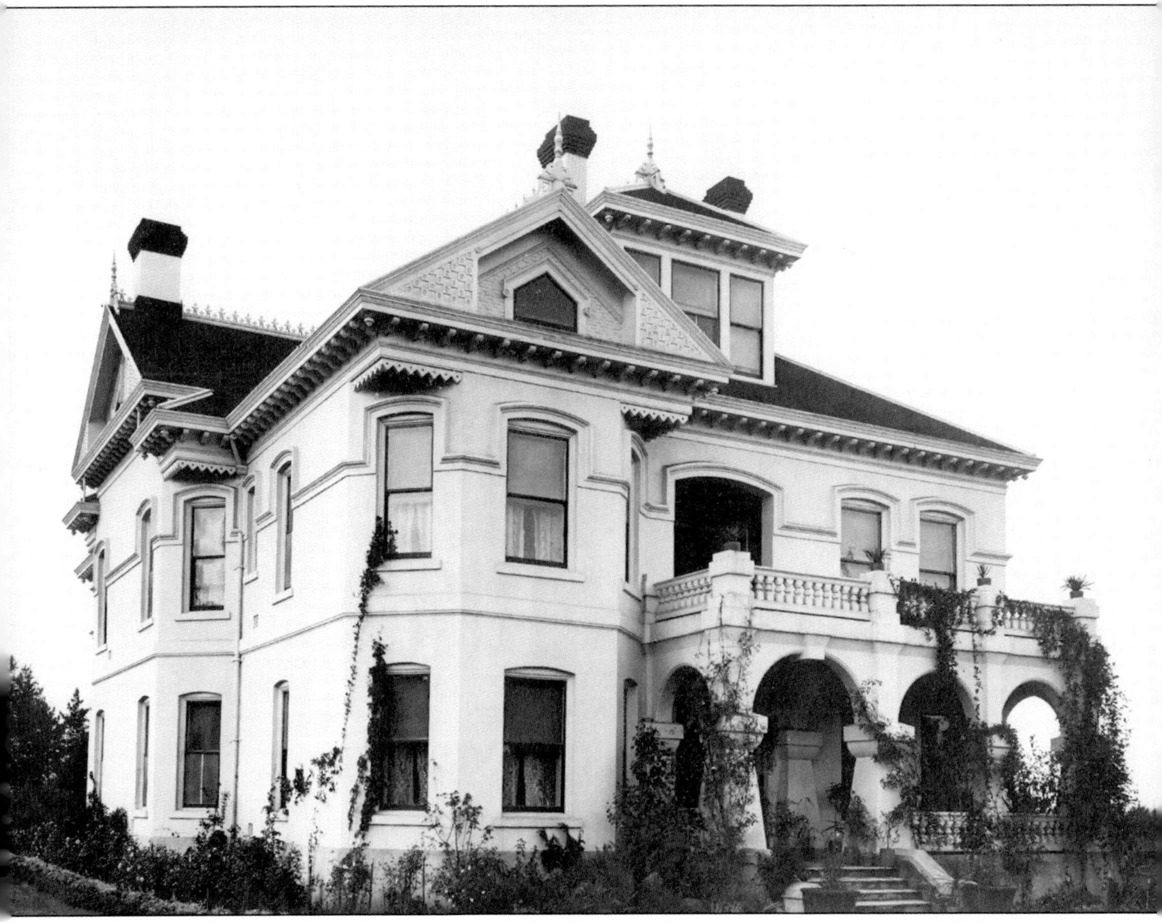

Napa architect Luther Turton designed this 18-room Queen Anne residence in 1898. It was the first superintendent's home; A.M. Gardner, L.F. Dozier, E.E. Stone, A.E. Osborne, and A.W. Horsholt, respectively, all lived there with their families. Dr. A.C. Matthews elected to live in the first assistant's home when Dr. Horsholt died in 1920. Thereafter, it became a manse, or manor house, for the professional staff and more recently a public relations office and volunteer center. (Courtesy NSH.)

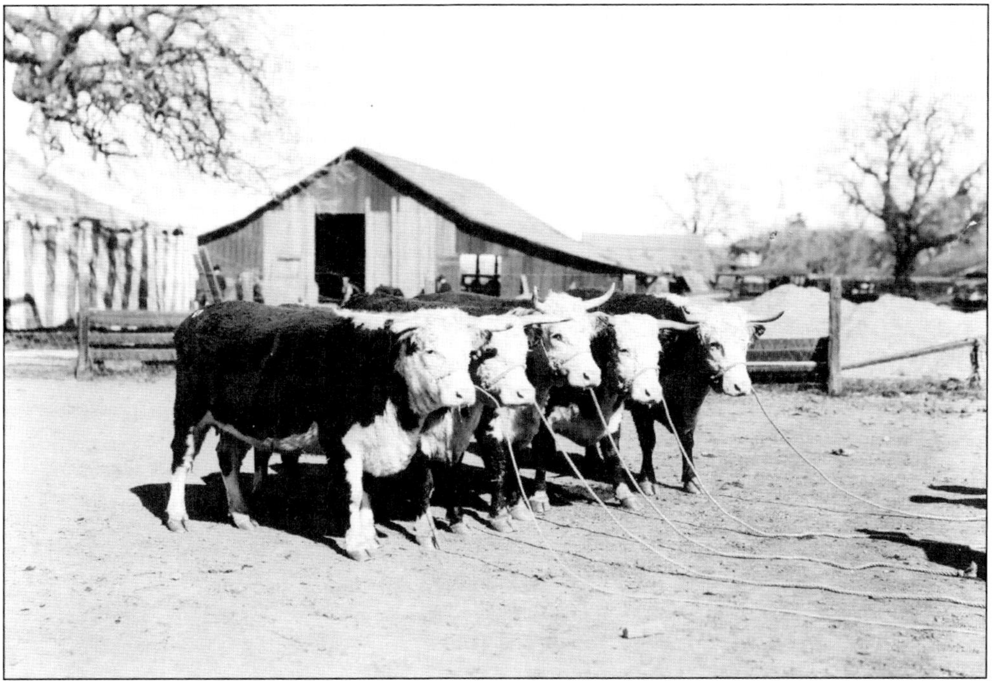

At times, the hospital dairy had up to 200 Holstein-Friesian cattle. It was the largest accredited herd in the state of California—and one of the best. The dairy won awards for its exceptional breeding and high butterfat content in milk nationwide. (Courtesy NCHS.)

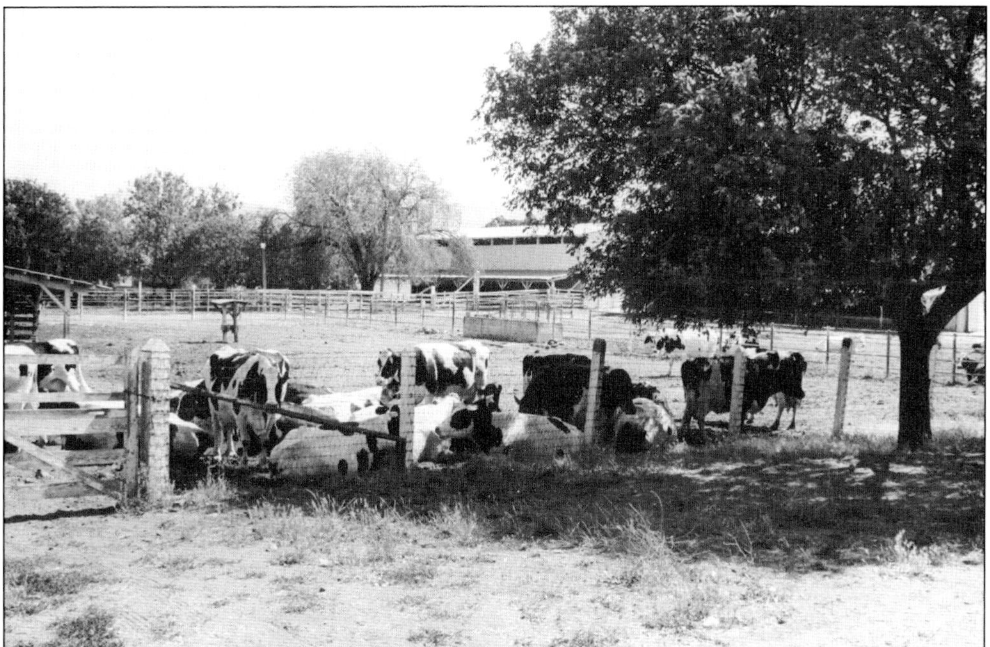

By 1916, the dairy consisted of 160 cows, producing about 10,000 gallons of milk monthly. New dairy barns, silos, and equipment were provided for $30,000. Under supervision, patients assisted in all facets of the operation. (Courtesy NSH.)

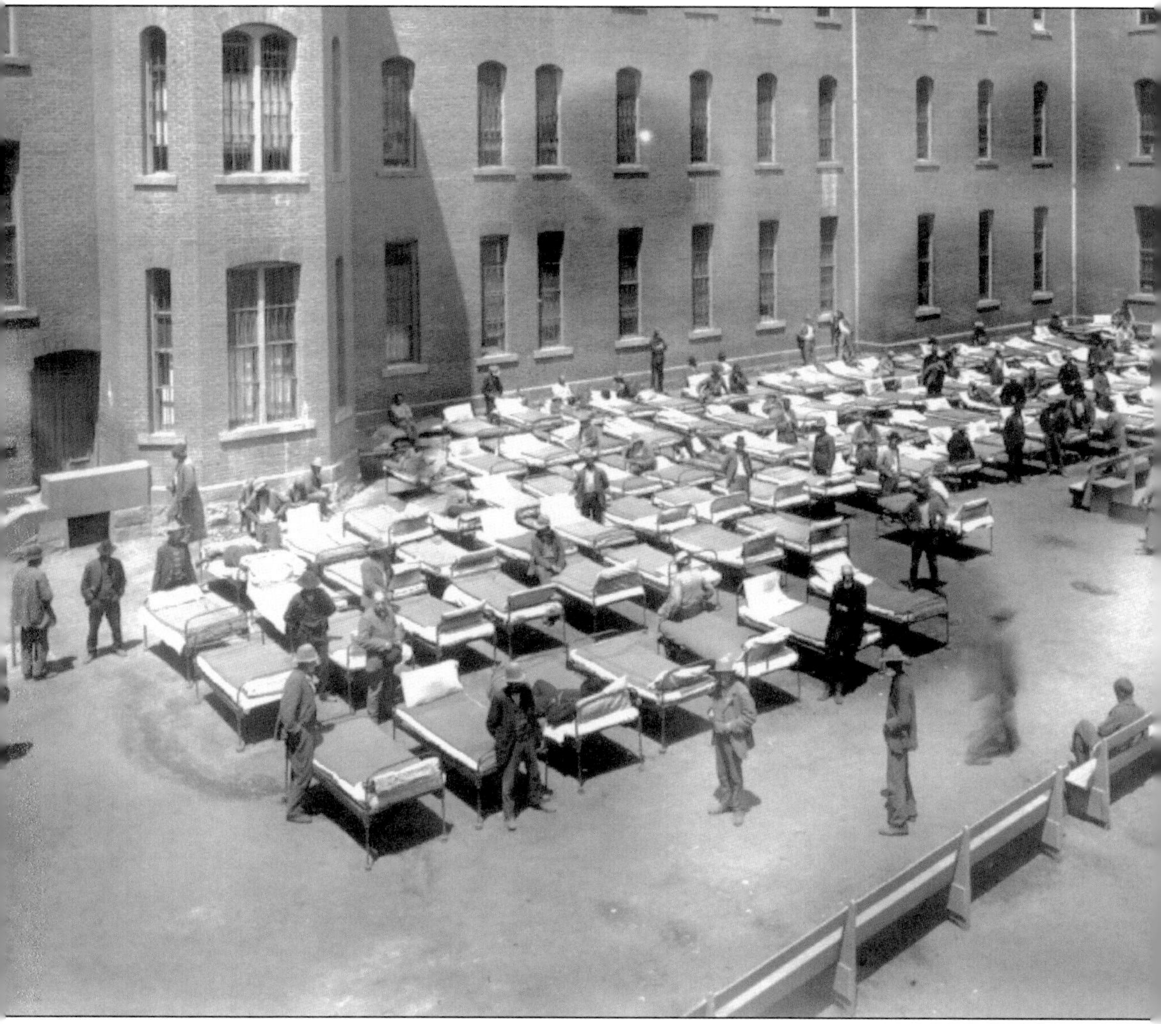

The beds of healthy patients were brought out to the Castle's courtyard to isolate them from the ill during an epidemic, possibly the 1918 flu. The *1916–1918 Biennial Report of the State Commission in Lunacy* stated that a shortage of nurses and attendants due to the war made the influenza pandemic difficult to handle despite taking proper precautions. At the height of the epidemic, there were 400 cases of the flu, including employees. (Courtesy NSH.)

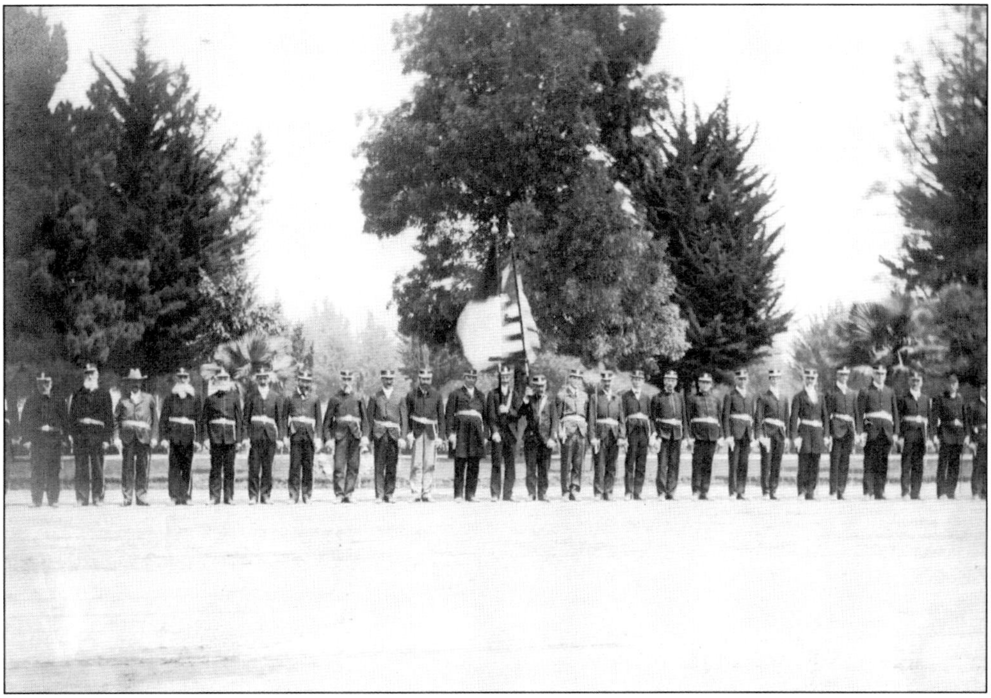

The patient drill team was a part of all parades and special events. (Courtesy NSH.)

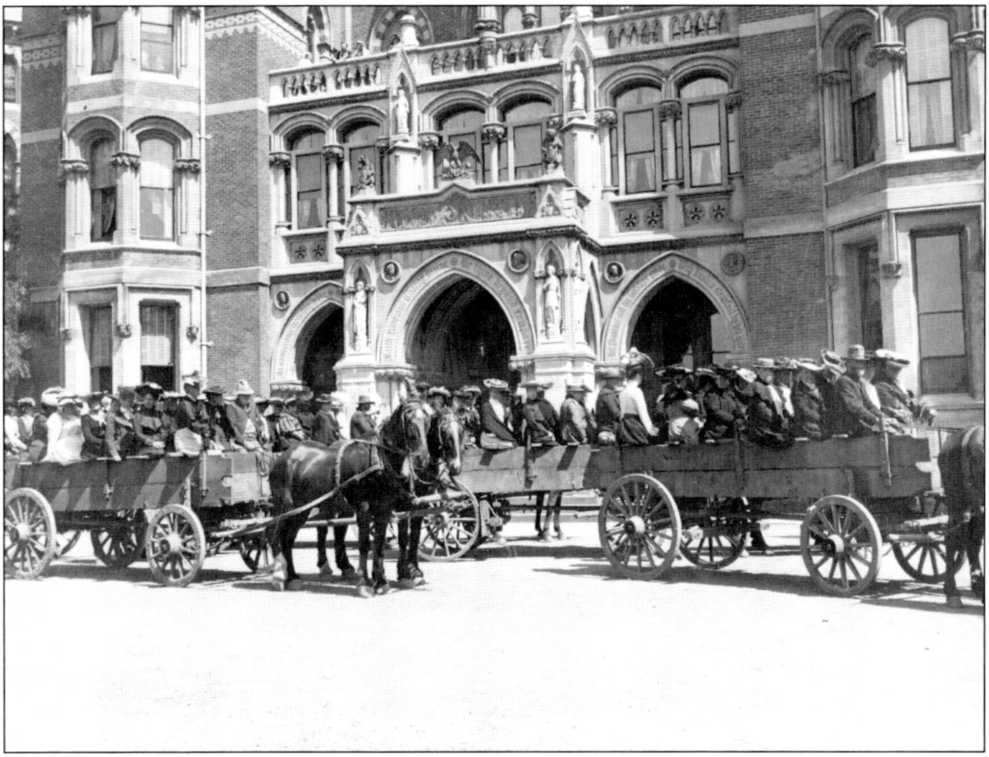

On a yearly basis, patients were loaded into wagons and taken into town for the circus and the Fourth of July Parade in Napa. (Courtesy NCHS.)

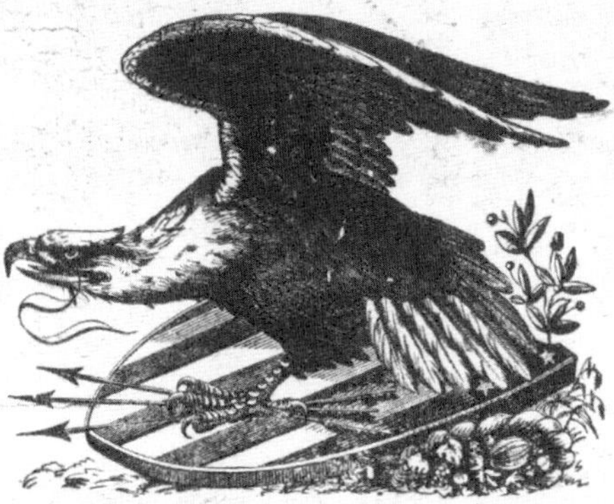

NAPA STATE HOSPITAL

Fourth of July
1908

Parade .... 8:30 A. M.
Song .... America
Overture .... Band
Oration .... Wm. Hudson Finch
Song .... Mrs. Josie Fair
Monologist .... Al. Yocum
Boxing Contest
Song .... Emil Casset
Song .... Miss Love
40 Yard Race .... Ladies
Sack Race .... Men
100 Yard Race .... Men
Greased Pole Climbing .... Men
Egg and Ladle Race .... Ladies
Shoe and Pea Race .... Men
Bucket Race .... Men
Three Legged Race .... Men
Fat Ladies' Race
Obstacle Race .... Men
Tug of War ....
Captains Fitzgerald and Melin
Nail Driving Contest .... Ladies
Ice Cream Contest Pie Eating Contest
Greased Pig
Dancing .... 9 A. M. to 1 P. M.

Among the events of the 1908 Fourth of July celebration were a parade, a speech by William Hudson Finch, a boxing contest, various races, greased-pole climbing, tug-of-war, an ice cream contest, a pie-eating contest, and dancing from 9:00 a.m. to 1:00 p.m. (Courtesy NCHS.)

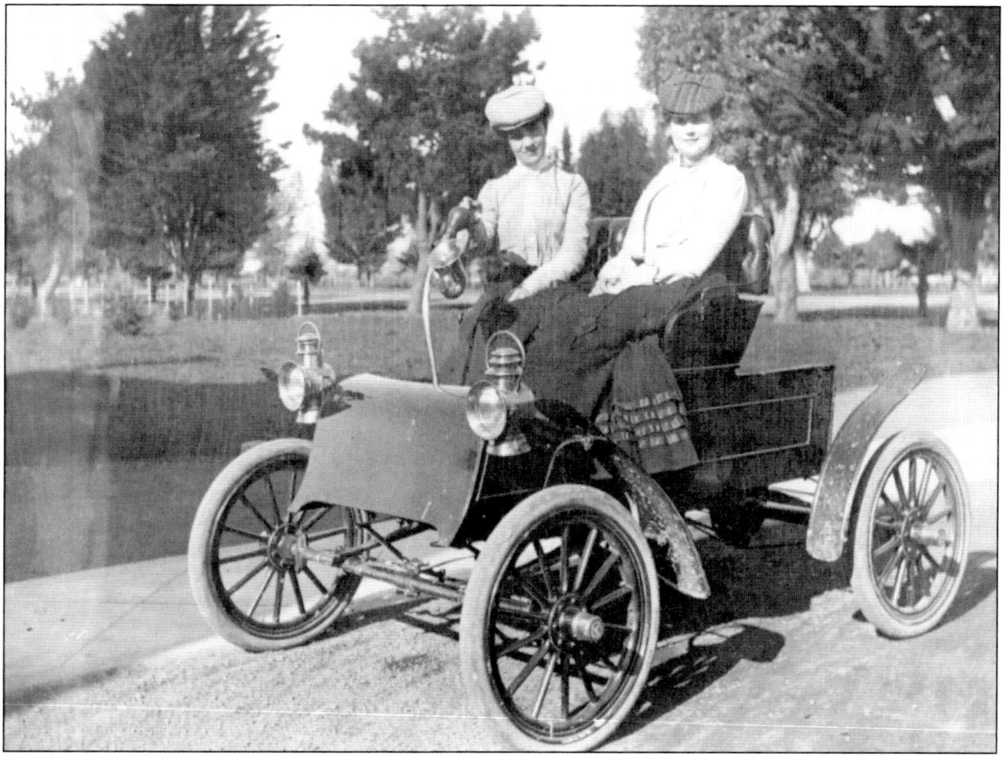

Pictured here are two doctors' wives enjoying a leisurely drive in an electric car. (Courtesy NSH.)

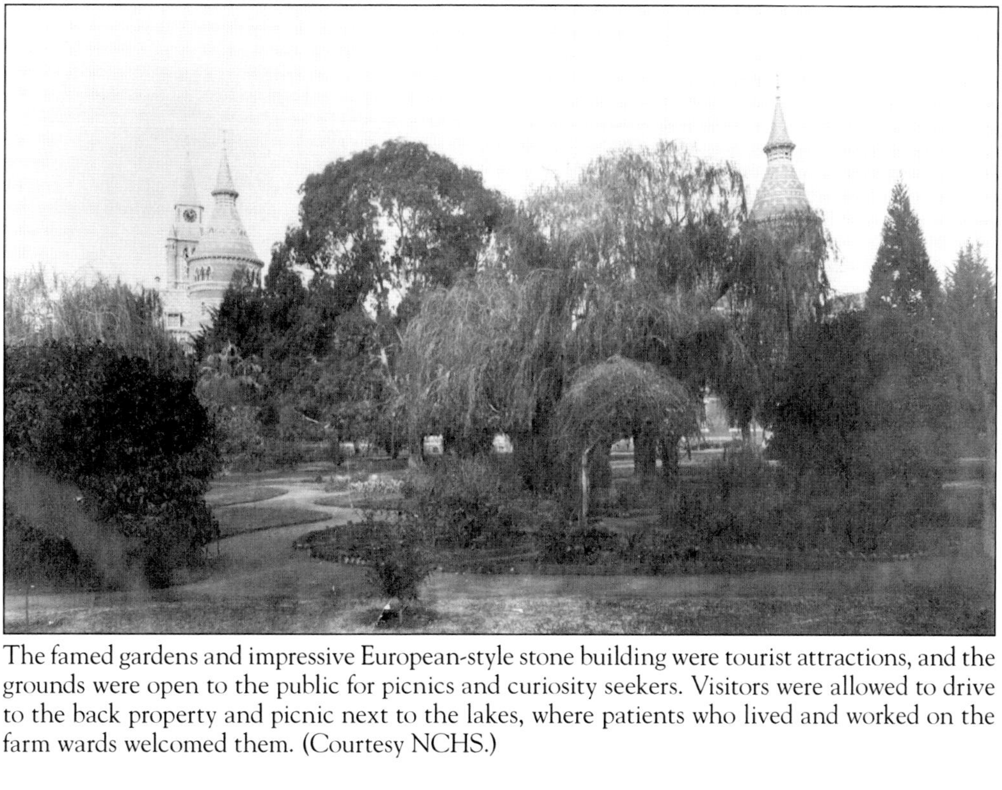

The famed gardens and impressive European-style stone building were tourist attractions, and the grounds were open to the public for picnics and curiosity seekers. Visitors were allowed to drive to the back property and picnic next to the lakes, where patients who lived and worked on the farm wards welcomed them. (Courtesy NCHS.)

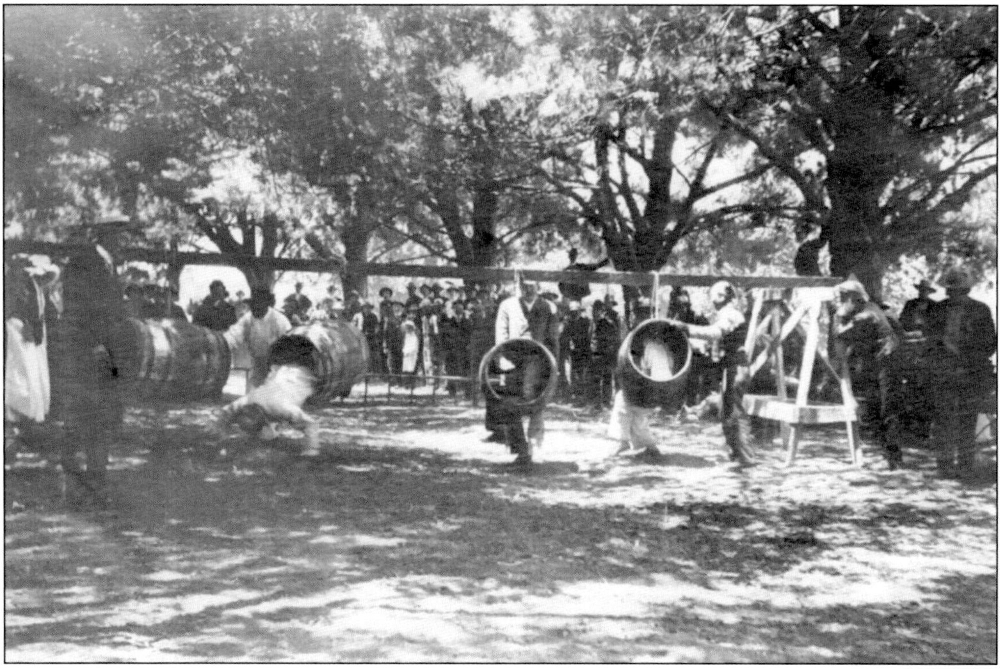

In addition to work therapy and exercises, patients were encouraged to attend dances and listen to music. Outdoor games, such as the one pictured here, were played with wine barrels. (Courtesy NSH.)

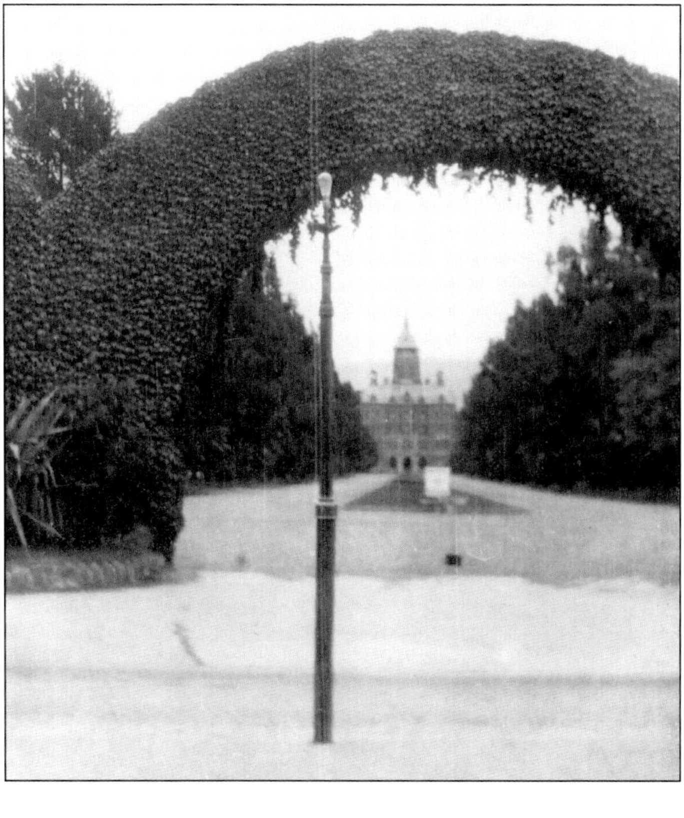

By 1910, the iron fence and gateway at the entrance had become so dilapidated that it was torn down, and a stone archway, covered with ivy in this photograph, was constructed. (Courtesy NCHS.)

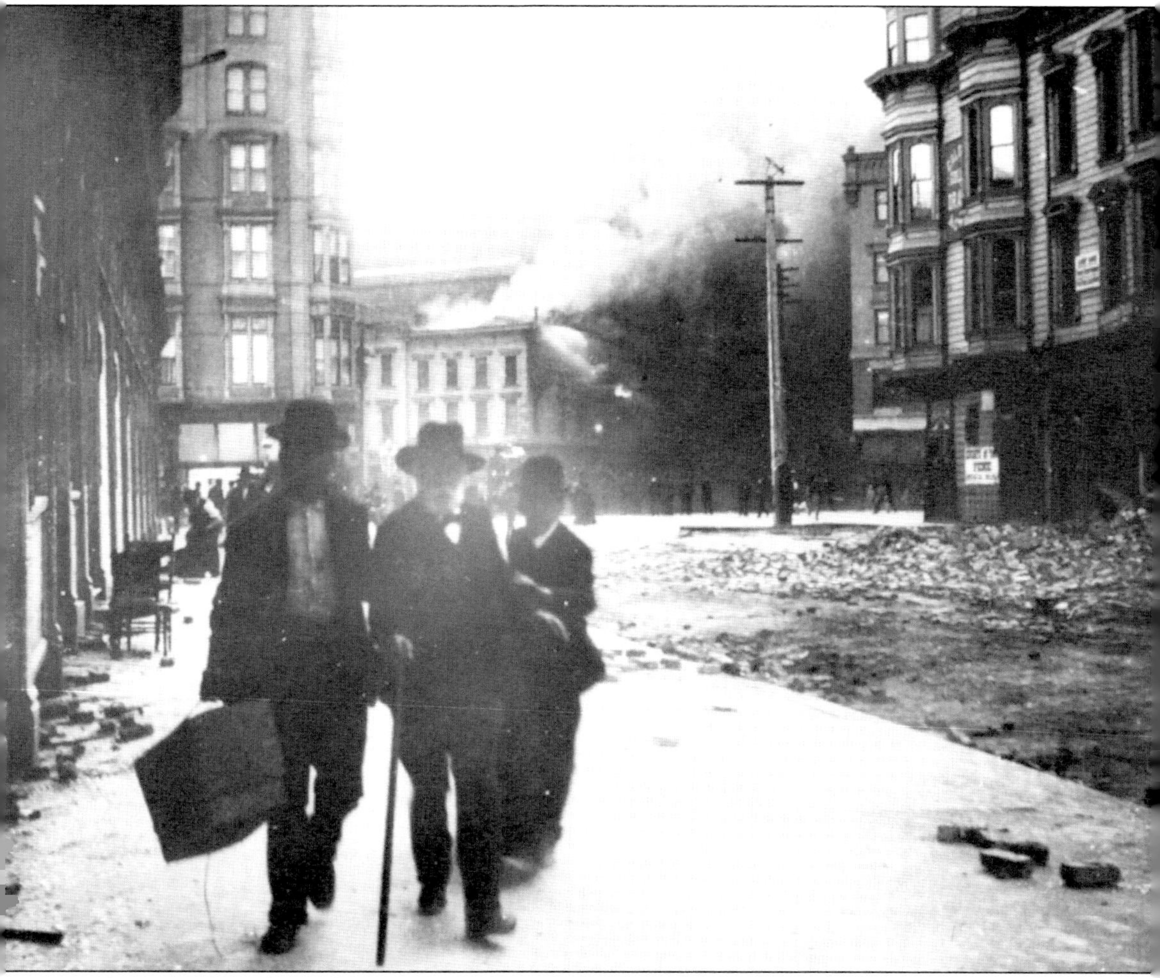

Carleton Watkins (center) is pictured here on April 18, 1906. He was an early photographer who captured Western landscapes, new cities, and industries. The 1906 earthquake and fire destroyed his studio and negatives. In 1909, his family committed him to the asylum for senile dementia; there, he is thought to be buried in an unmarked grave on the grounds. (Courtesy Bancroft Library.)

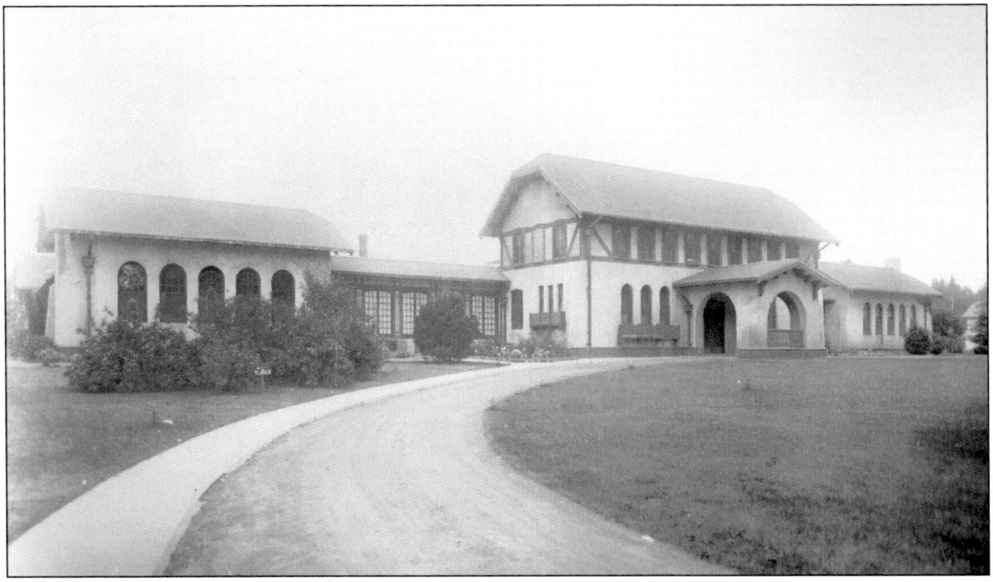

In response to overcrowding and evidence that larger institutions were equipped solely for custodial care and consequently could not adequately treat or cure patients, the state began adopting what was then known as the Cottage Hospital Model. The B Ward, also known as the admission unit, was built in 1913 and was called the Acute Quiet Hospital. It was the facility for primarily hydrotherapy treatments. The left wing was male, and the right wing was female, with offices located above the entrance. There was a corridor in the center with treatment rooms, allowing for enclosed patios on either side. (Courtesy CSA.)

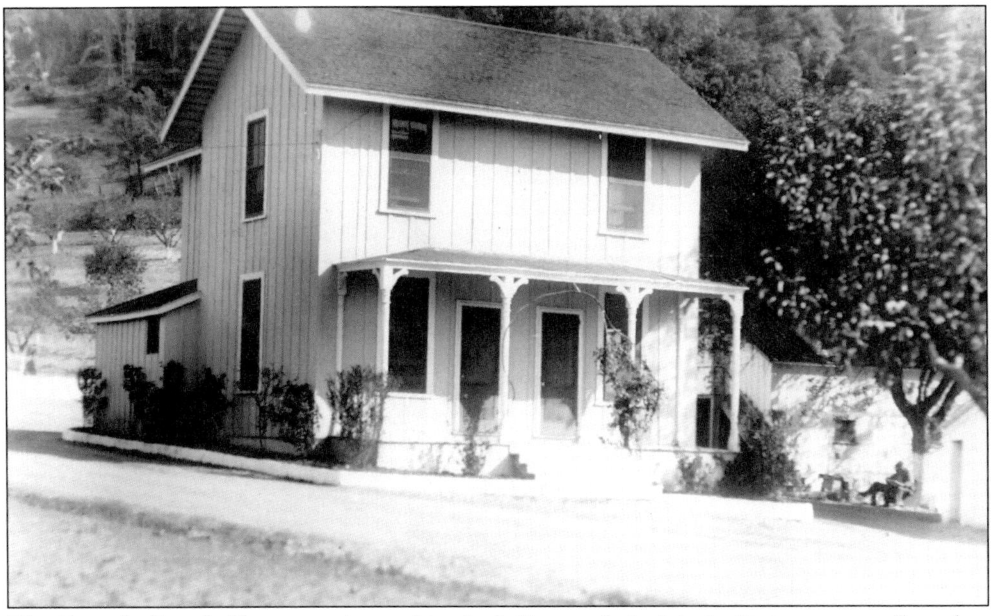

The Coombs Ranch House was located in the hills near Lake Marie. Patients were allowed to build their own cabins and sleeping shelters across Lake Marie Creek. More farmworkers needed sleeping quarters, and more beds were always needed in the Castle. A large cabin beyond the creek was built by a Spanish War veteran, who welcomed visitors when they arrived in their horse-drawn carriages. Once there, they would stop and enjoy a picnic by the lake. (Courtesy NSH.)

Two

WORK THERAPY 1916–1918

Work therapy programs were largely successful. The asylum was self-sustaining and sold surplus produce and milk to other institutions. Imola was the largest state institution and largest employer in Napa. Numerous patients benefitted from the relative security and predictability of asylum life. The state could not, unfortunately, keep up with rising admissions and declining discharges in all of their asylums—a sure sign that perhaps moral treatment and dependence on the institution was not an effective solution for the long term.

As the 20th century dawned, and as psychiatry matured, new theories were developed with the hope of providing quicker cures for patients who were crowded into recreation rooms and often sleeping on mattresses in hallways, attics, and basements. Treatments focused on the mind-body connection, with hydrotherapy, sterilization, and malaria fever therapy becoming the most prevalent in the 1910s and 1920s. According to Joel Braslow in *Mental Ills and Bodily Cures*, California led the nation in sterilizing psychiatric patients and in 1921 had performed 80 percent of all state hospital patient sterilizations in the United States. In the 1930s, electroshock therapy and psychosurgery were widely practiced on "chronic" or "hopeless" cases and often on troubled adolescents. Both treatments were controversial, sometimes even lethal, yet they were considered to be medical treatments with the intent to prevent relapses or a lifetime spent in an institution.

The Department of Institutions was formed in 1921 to modernize treatments and alter viewpoints on mental illness. Napa Asylum for the Insane changed its name to Napa State Hospital in 1924, as did all of the California state asylums.

(1497) The men are first taught to march and to keep time.

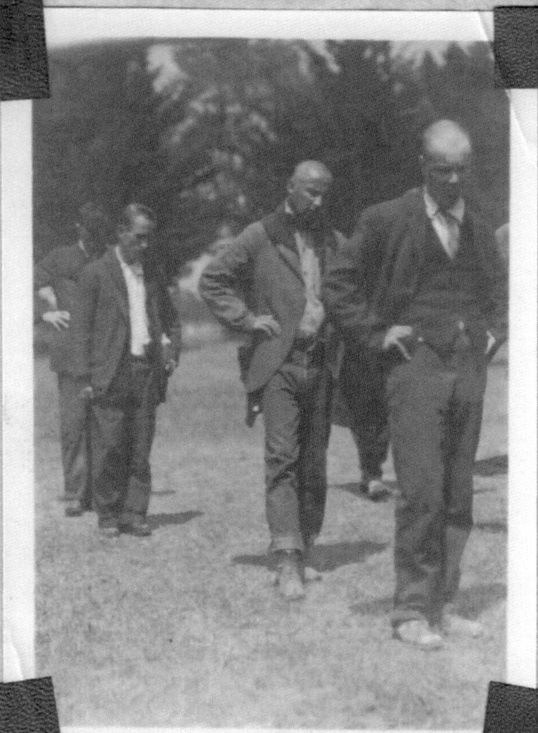

(1499)

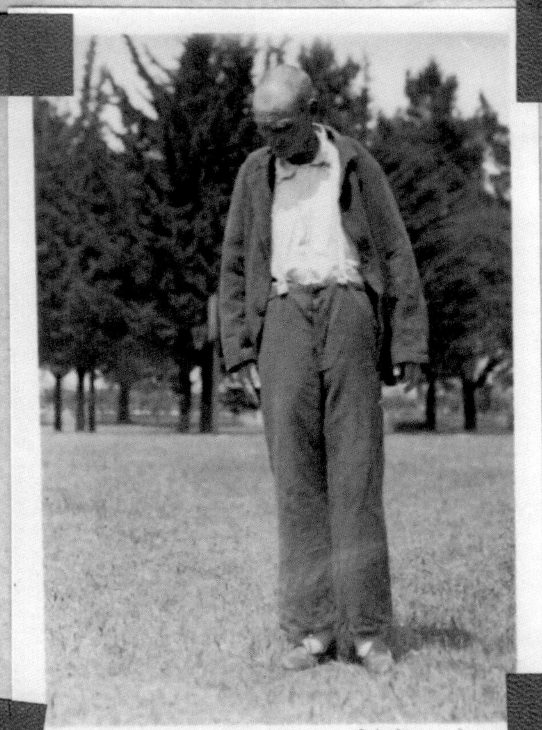

(1500)

The above pictures show some of the patients shortly after their entrance to the class of exercises.

The following 17 photographs, labeled as "William A. Locarini, Attorney at Law," were taken as evidence for an unknown case. Its intent was to defend the effectiveness of the asylum's work therapy program. The original captions are provided under each photograph. Also included are before-and-after photographs. (All photographs in this chapter courtesy NCHS.)

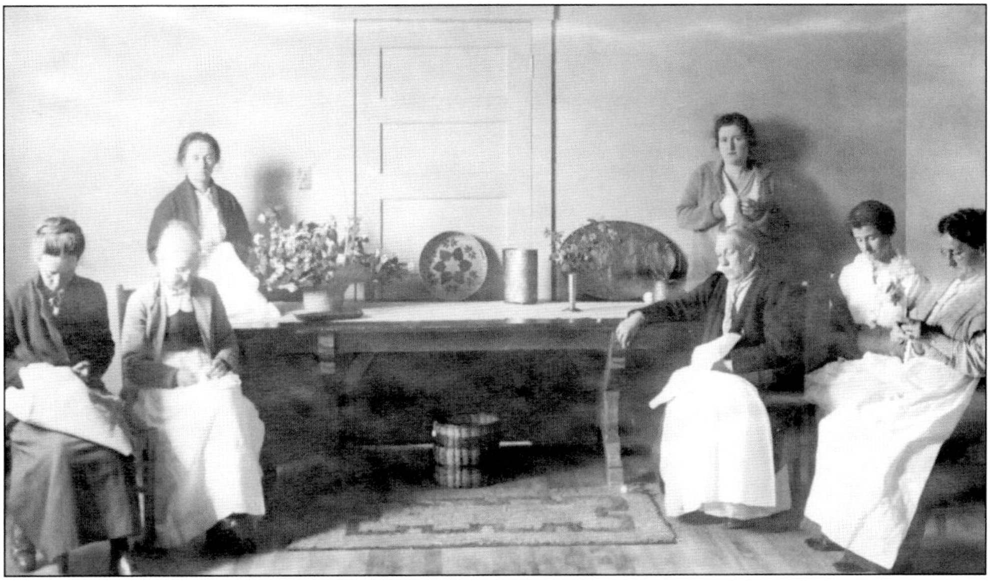

"We have six work rooms. The first room, which is 8 x 18 feet is used for exhibition purposes. The second room, which is 18 x 20 feet is used for needlework, crocheting, and fancy work, accommodating about eight patients."

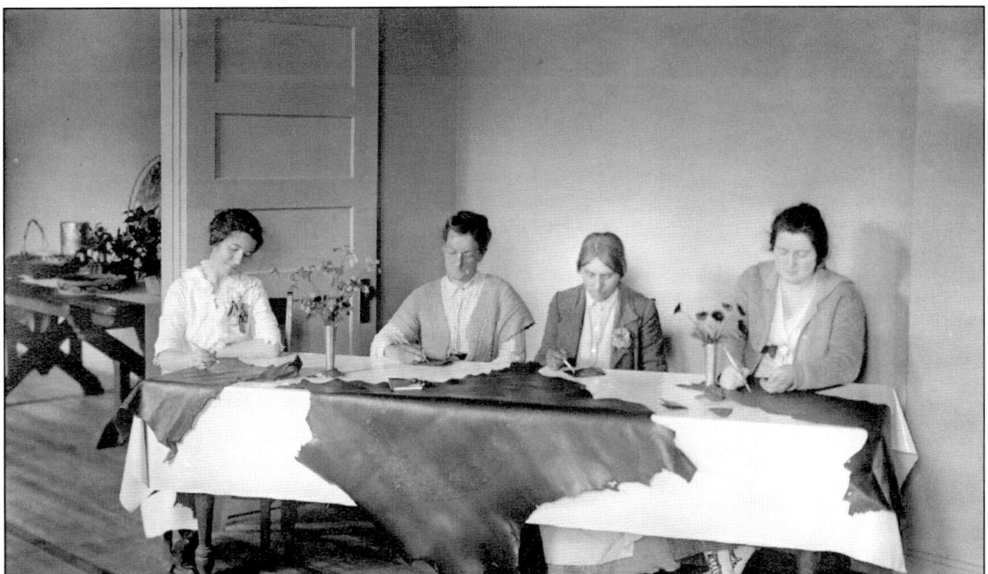

"Between the second and third work rooms are folding doors which allow the two rooms to be thrown together for small parties. The third room is 18 x 20 feet and is used for work on tooled leather, wood carving, and lace weaving, accommodating five patients."

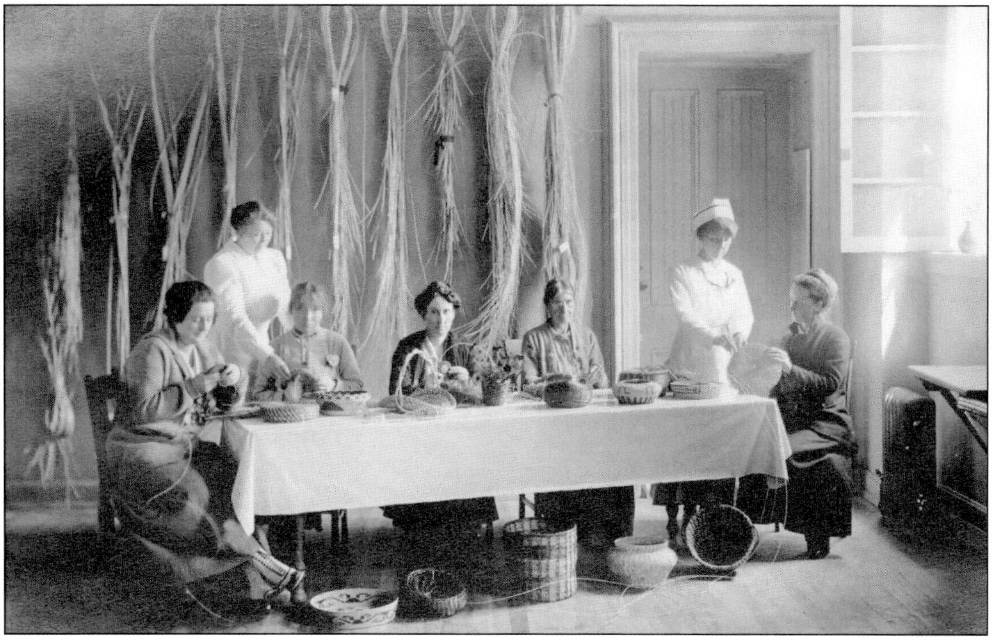

“In the fourth room which is 18 x 24 feet, is the class in basketry. All sorts of baskets are made: Indian, reed, corn, husk, pine needle, and native grasses. In this room we have eight patients working.”

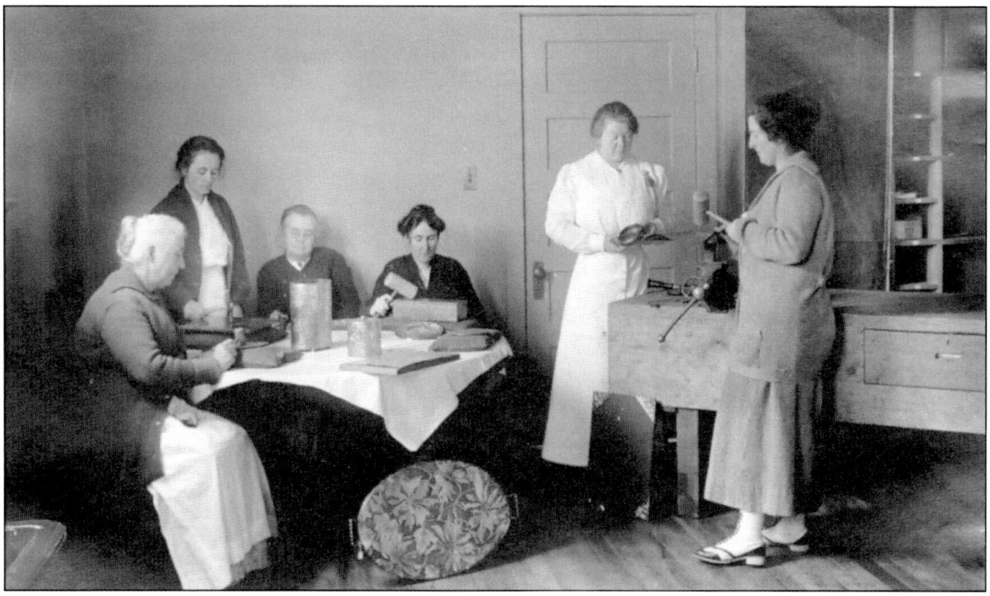

“In the fifth room, which is 20 x 40 feet, we have our rug looms, linen looms, bench for copper and brass and table for clay work. Ten patients may be accommodated here.”

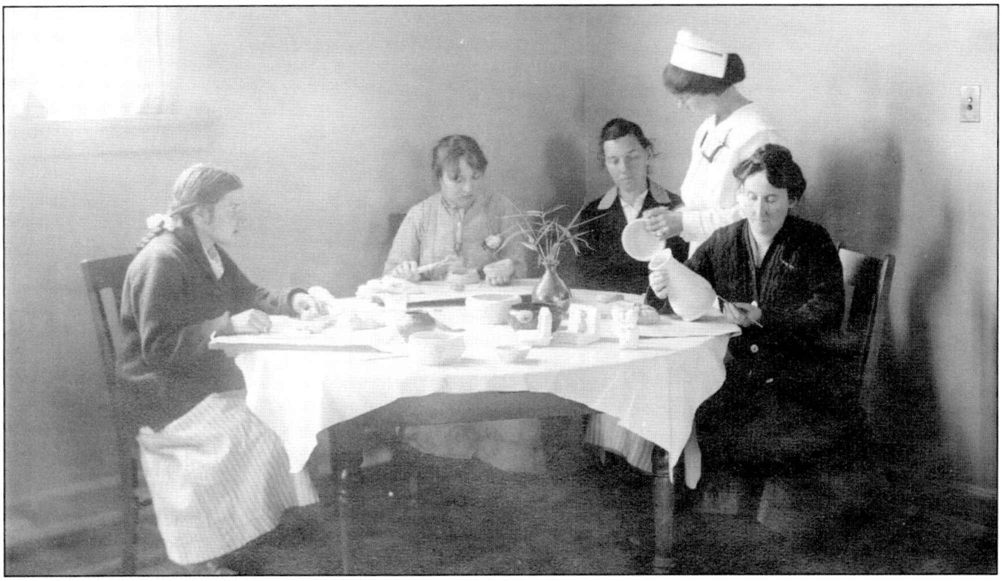

"Dementia praecox clay work." Patients were expected to labor at least four hours a day, especially the women, who tended to have skills like cooking, cleaning, and sewing that were useful to the asylum.

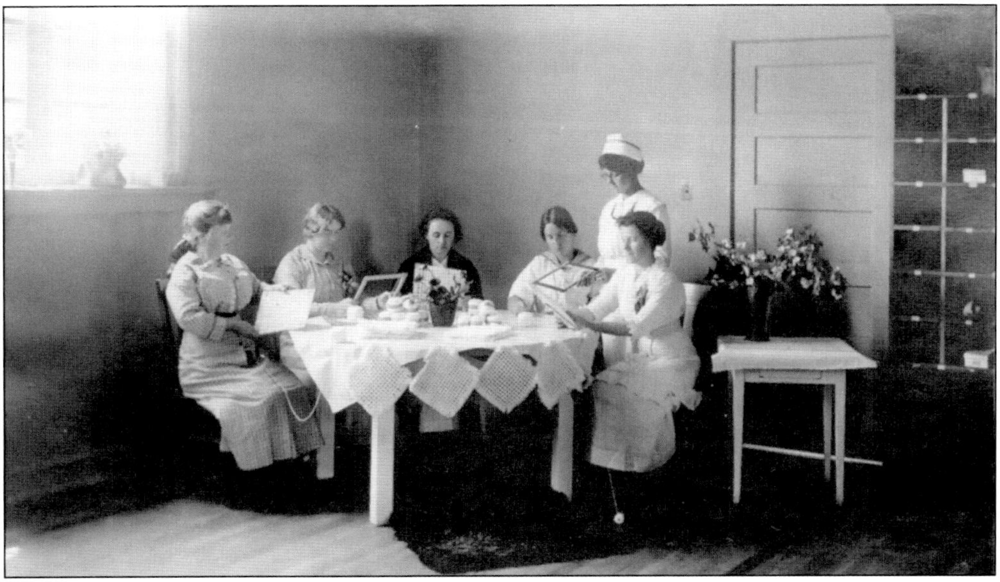

"Dementia praecox—colonial mats. The stock room and office is off the large work room. All of the rooms are bright, attractive and cheerful, the furnishings blending harmoniously with the walls and hangings, which are a rich tan color. We keep in these rooms at all times a profusion of flowers. Note. We are unable to give the economic saving to the hospital by occupational work as we have been working a little over one year."

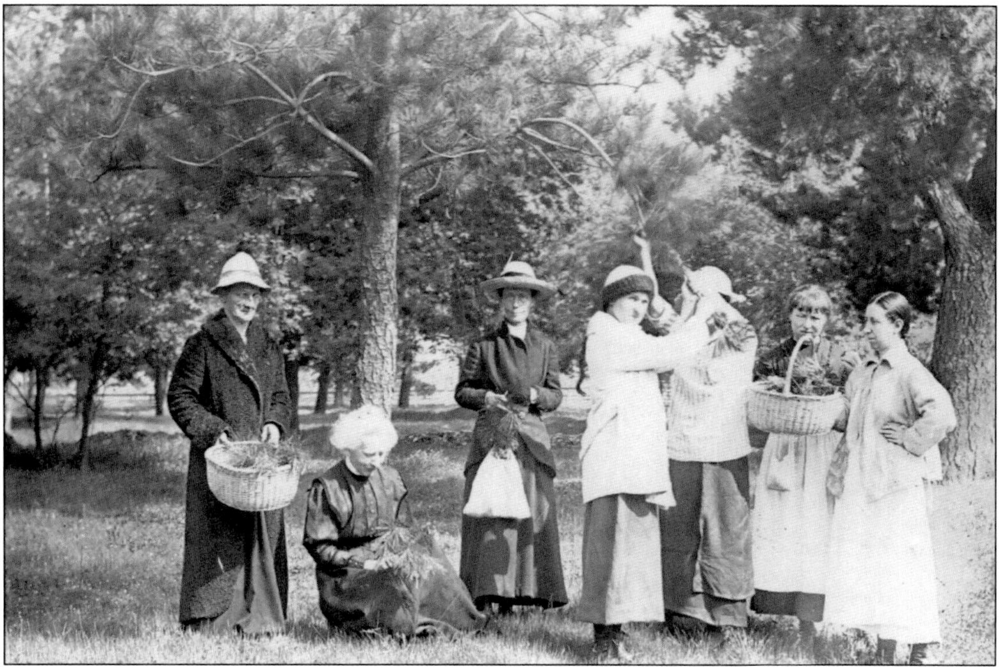

"Work therapy class gathering pine needles on the hospital grounds."

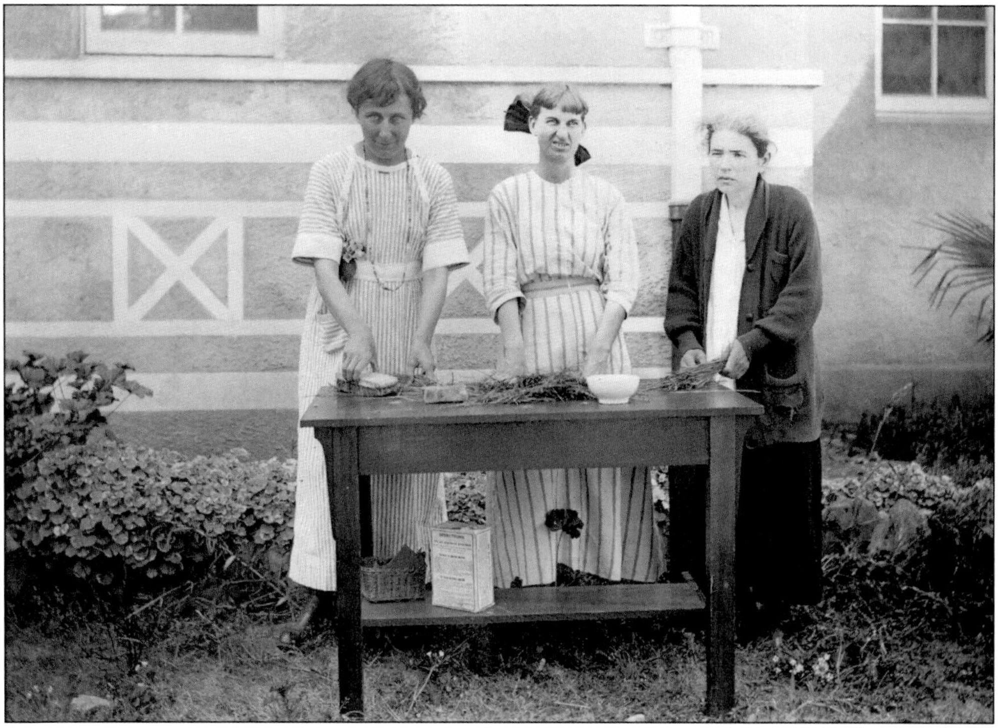

"Patients preparing pine needles."

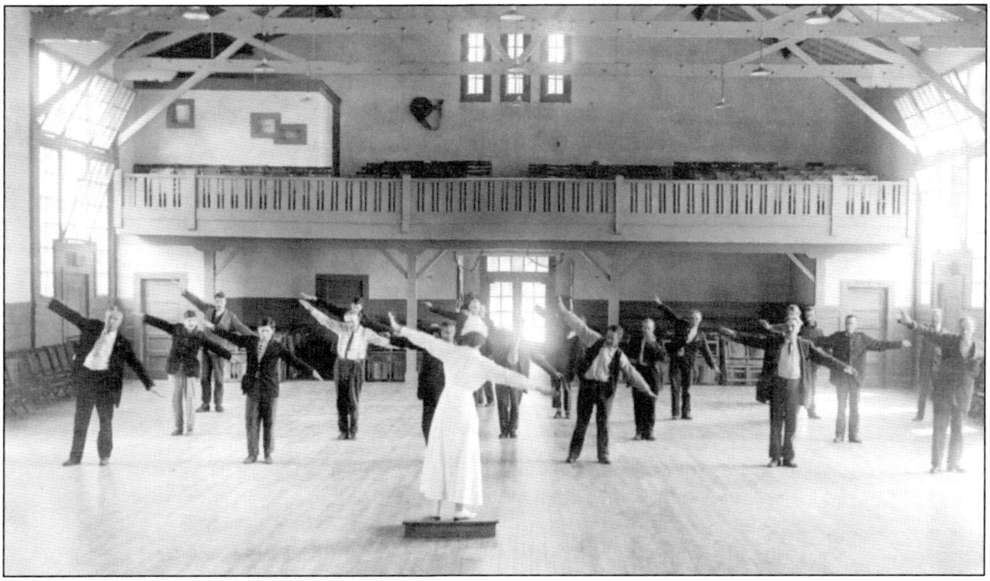

"The dementia praecox men are first taught to follow in a simple march to stirring music, to form into simple drills and setting-up exercises."

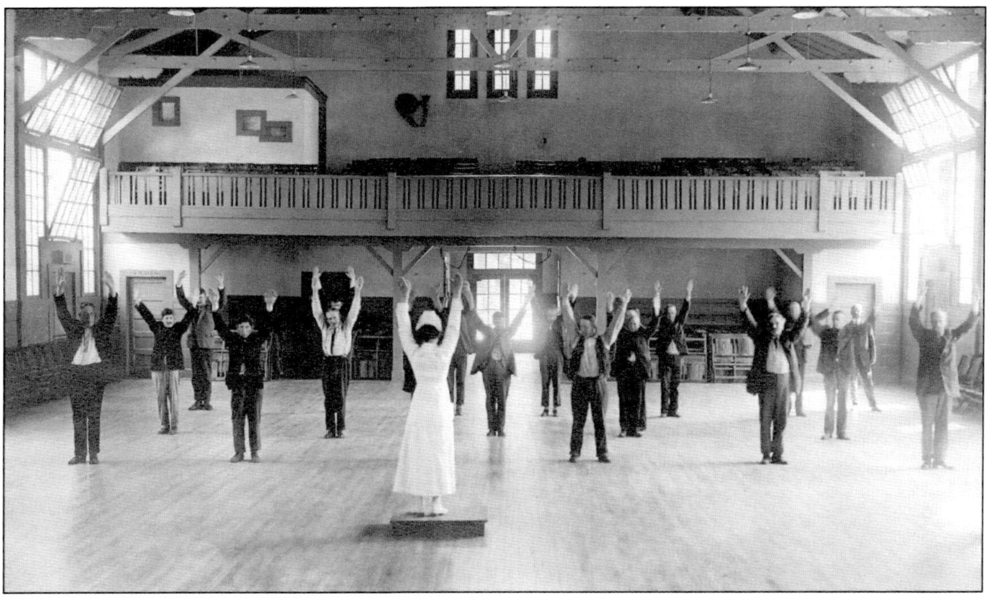

"An attendant is always present to assist the instructress as many of the patients have to be started each time the exercise changes. After some time they are able to follow and begin each exercise if spoken to and gradually succeed in watching and following the teacher's example."

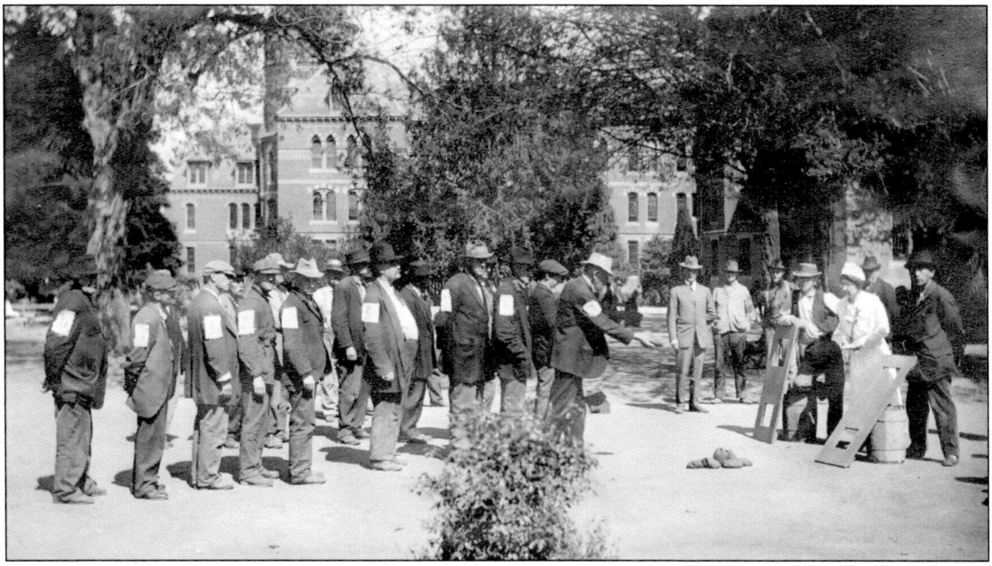

"As these patients gradually become better they are interested in games which are played in the yards. Here they are playing a bean bag game."

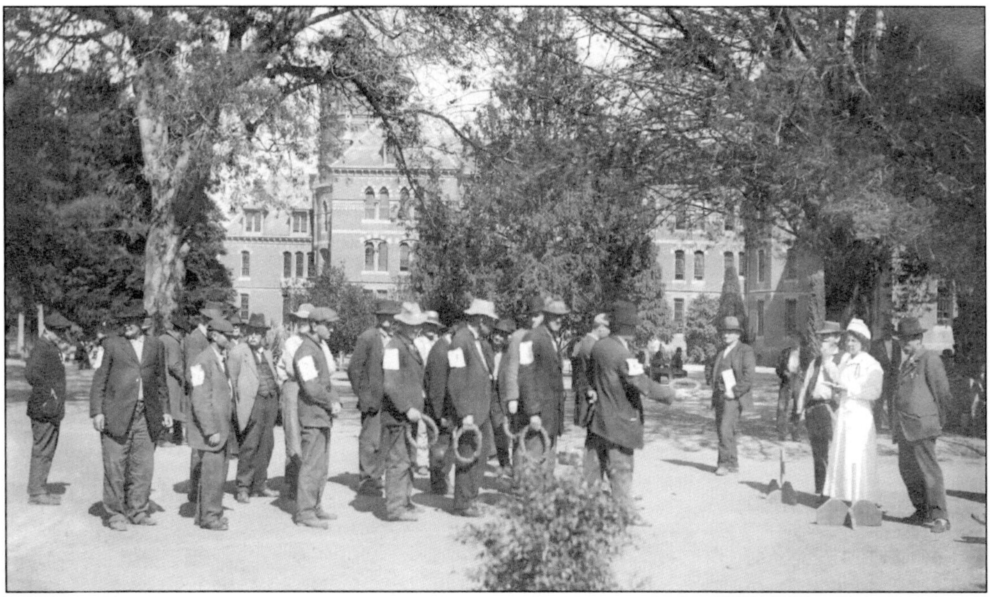

"Here they are playing a rope quoit game."

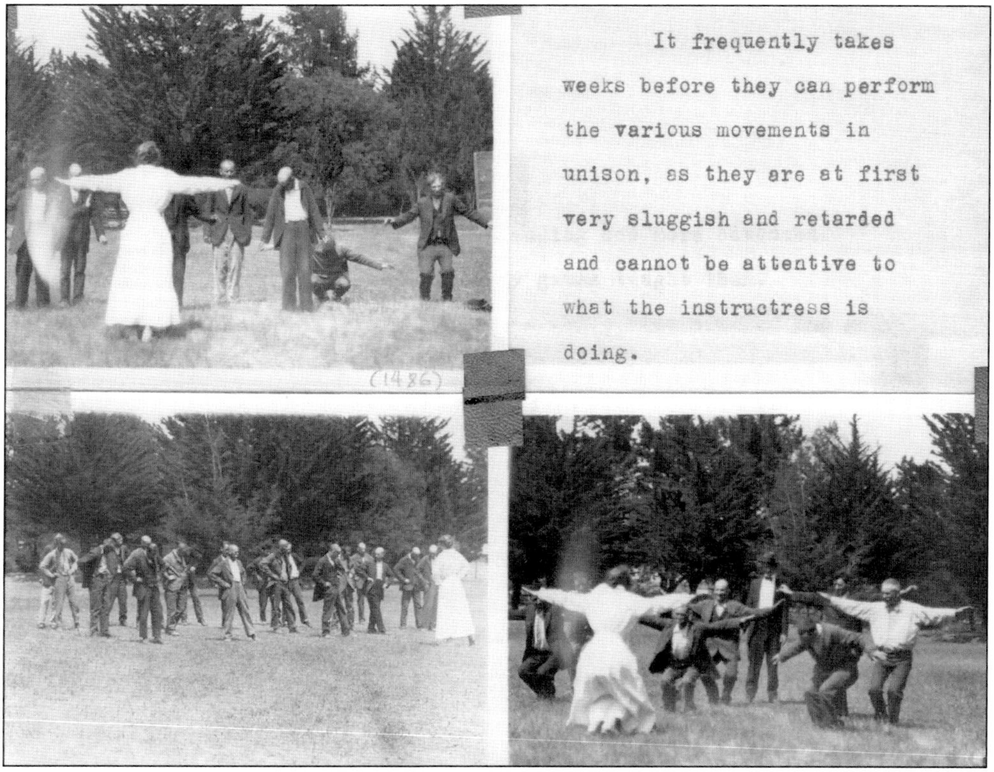

"It frequently takes weeks before they can perform the various movements in unison, as they are at first very sluggish and retarded and cannot be attentive to what the instructress is doing."

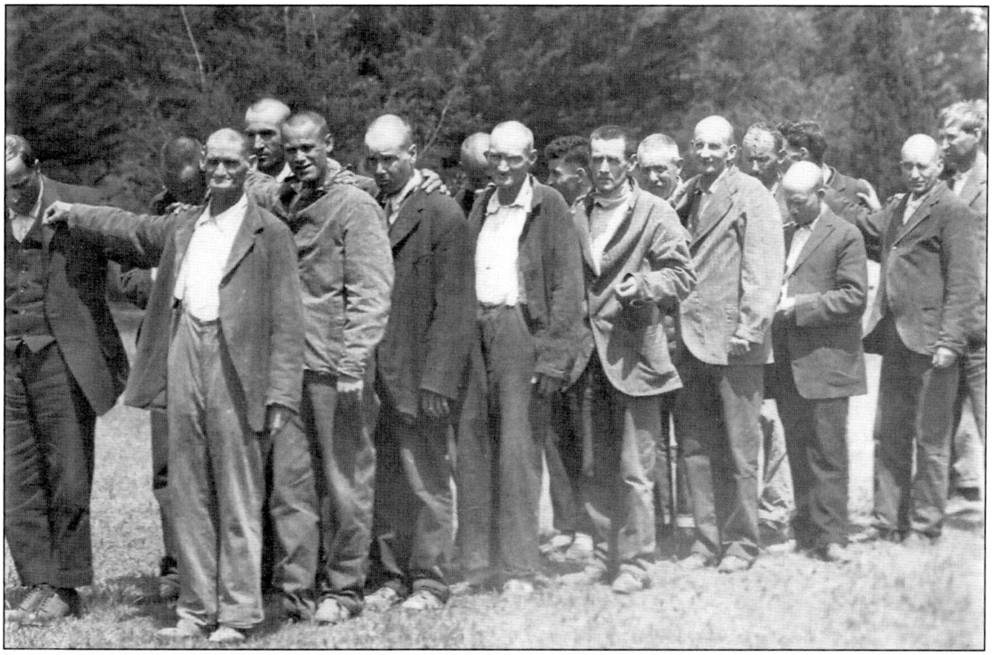

"These classes are held out-of-doors and in the gymnasium—the music for the exercises is furnished by some of the patients. The men are first taught to march and keep time."

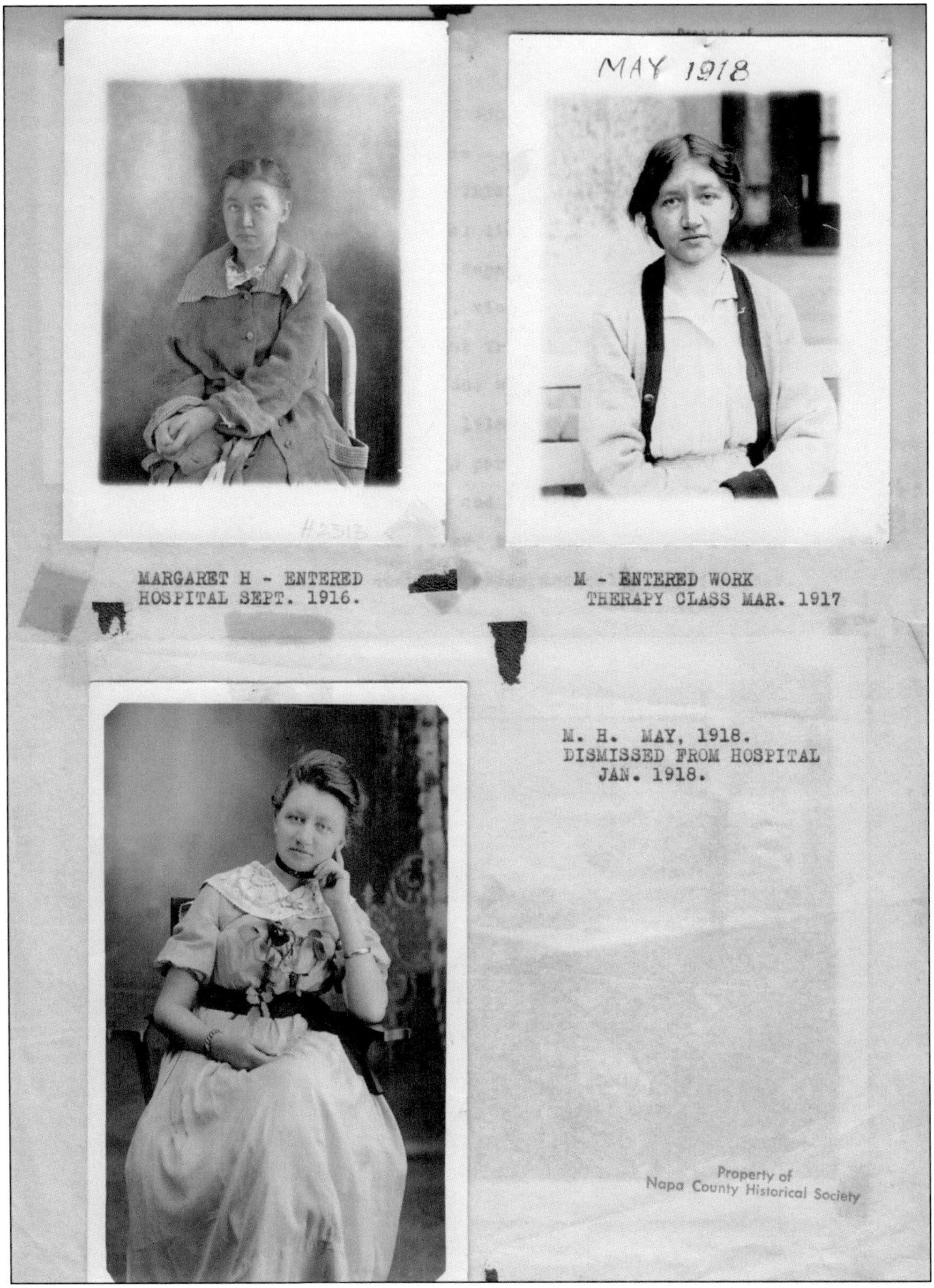

"Margaret H [above left]—Entered hospital Sept. 1916. . . . M [above right]—Entered work therapy class Mar. 1917. . . . M. H. May [below left], 1918. Dismissed from hospital Jan. 1918."

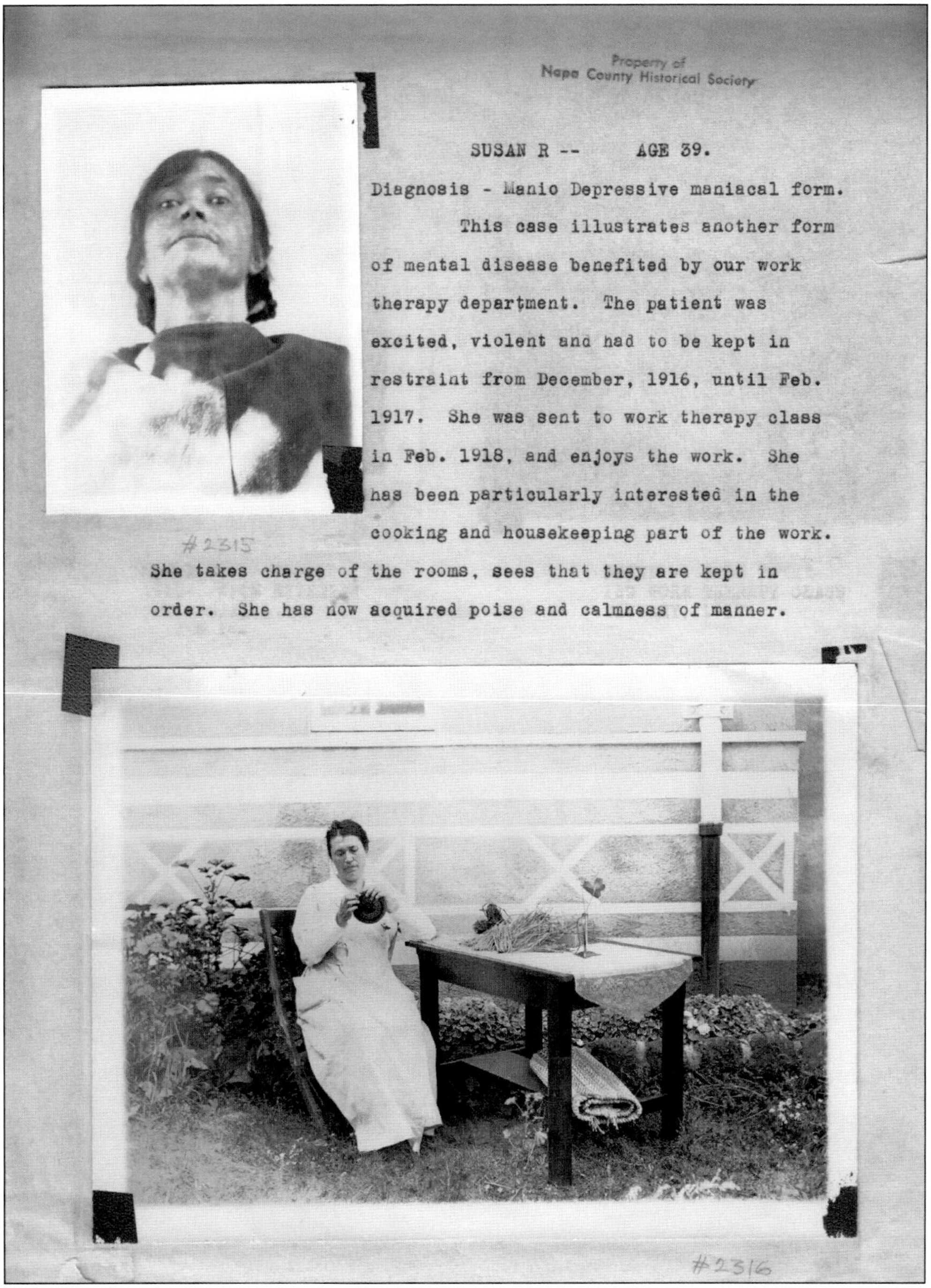
Property of
Napa County Historical Society

SUSAN R -- AGE 39.

Diagnosis - Manio Depressive maniacal form.

This case illustrates another form of mental disease benefited by our work therapy department. The patient was excited, violent and had to be kept in restraint from December, 1916, until Feb. 1917. She was sent to work therapy class in Feb. 1918, and enjoys the work. She has been particularly interested in the cooking and housekeeping part of the work. She takes charge of the rooms, sees that they are kept in order. She has now acquired poise and calmness of manner.

#2315

#2316

"Susan R—Age 39. Diagnosis—Manic Depressive maniacal form. This case illustrates another form of mental disease benefited by our work therapy department. The patient was excited, violent and had to be kept in restraint from December, 1916, until Feb. 1917. She was sent to work therapy class in Feb. 1918, and enjoys the work. She has been particularly interested in the cooking and housekeeping part of the work. She takes charge of the rooms, sees that they are kept in order. She has now acquired poise and calmness of manner."

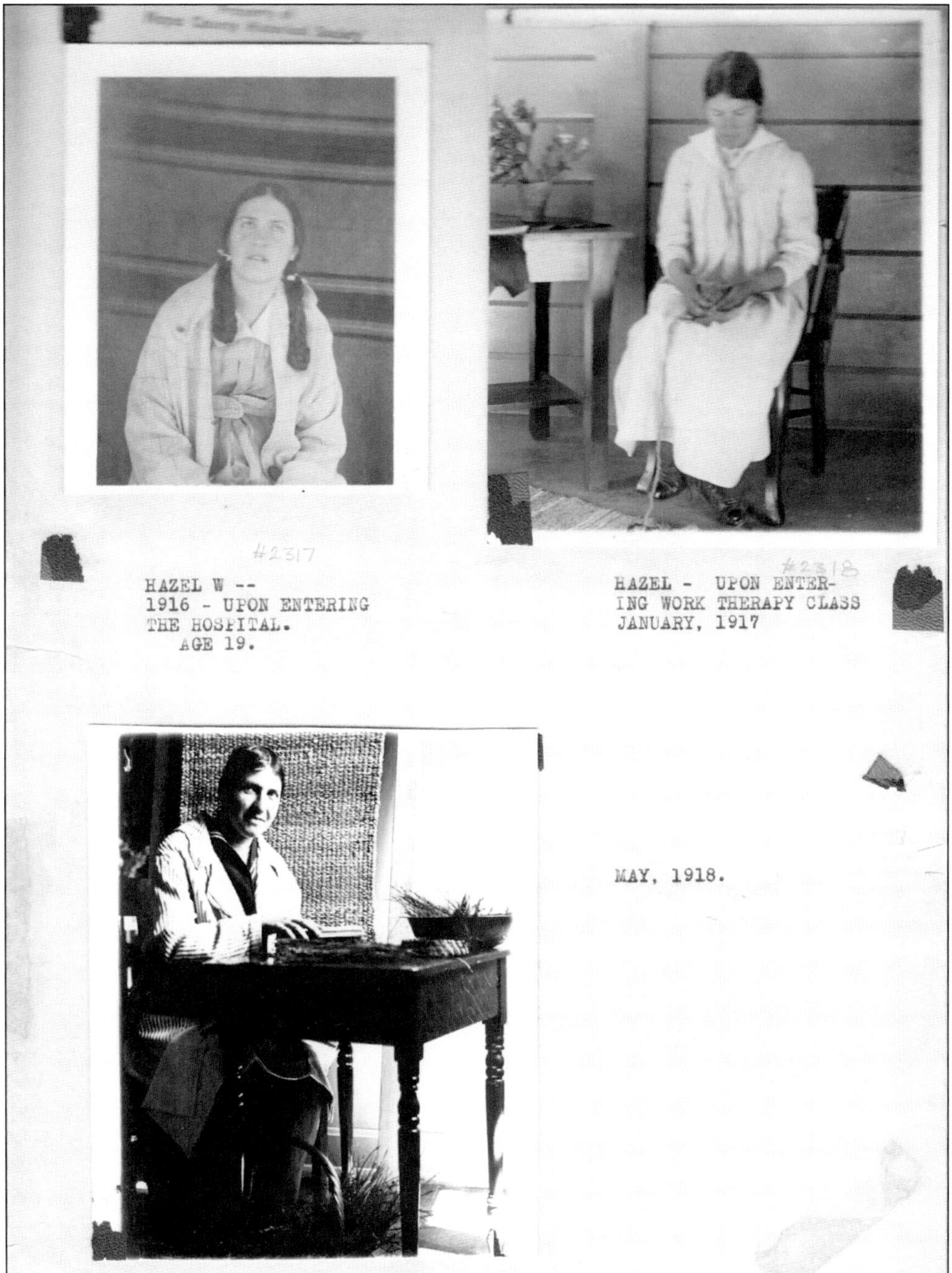

"Hazel W [above left]—1916—Upon entering the hospital. Age 19. . . . Hazel [above right]—Upon entering work therapy class January, 1917. . . . May [below left], 1918."

Three

From Insane Asylum to State Hospital 1922–1954

As overcrowded conditions in the deteriorating Castle building continued to make caring for patients a daily struggle, World War II required the hospital to assist with the war effort. Plans to demolish the Castle and build a new facility were postponed due to a shortage of construction materials.

To Napans, it was still known as Imola—an integral part of the community. It was a home to countless families who lived and worked there for two or three generations. Cindi Hummer's grandparents, parents, and uncle provided over 100 years of state service. She recalls that it was a close-knit, social community. Her mother worked in the Receiving Unit for 25 years and ran the Imola Broadcasting System, which aired music and news. Her father was a full-time fireman for 38 years. The children played on huge swing sets near the hospital entrance and enjoyed exploring the property, which was their back yard. Every Christmas Day, Santa's sleigh was pulled by the chief's truck around the grounds, with her dad, Vernon Nowlin, dressed as Santa Claus.

Some lamented the loss of the regal Castle building in 1950, for which many had a sense of pride. Others rejoiced, hoping that modern elevators, better water pressure, and smaller wards would improve working and living conditions.

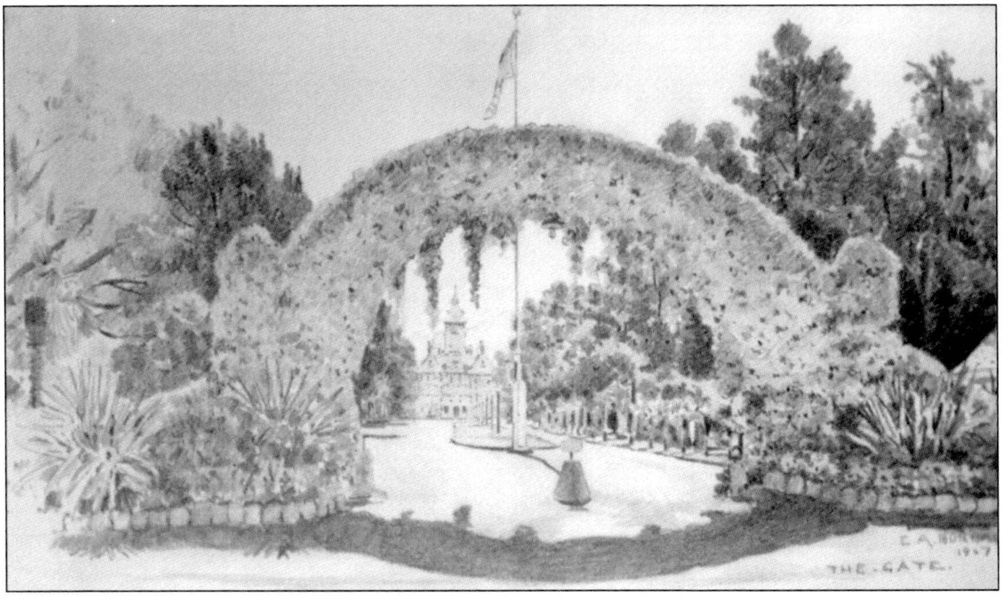

E.A. Burbank was an American artist who sketched and painted more than 1,200 portraits of Native Americans from 125 tribes. As an adult, Burbank was diagnosed with bipolar disorder, known then as "manic depression." He was voluntarily committed and spent nearly 20 years in Imola from 1917 to 1936. (Courtesy NCHS.)

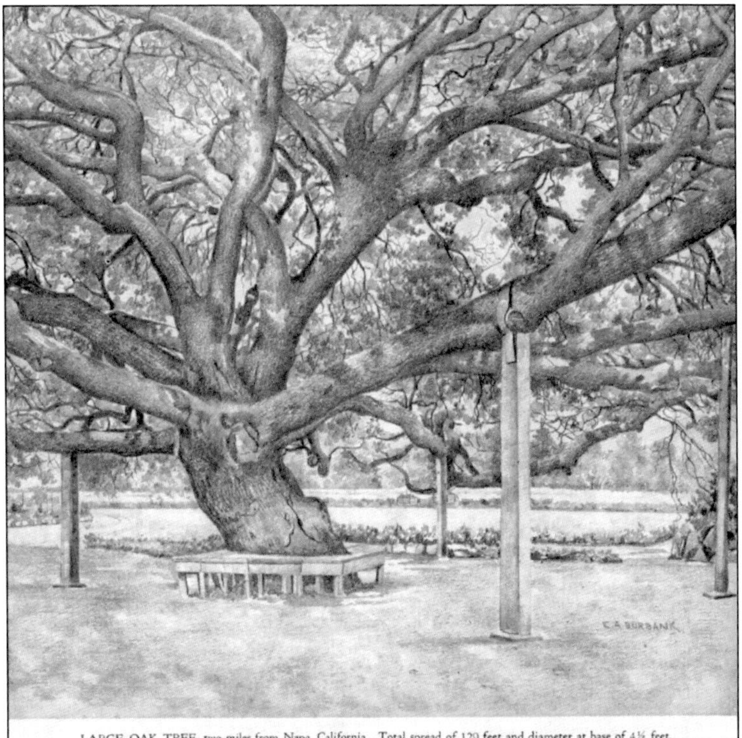

LARGE OAK TREE, two miles from Napa, California. Total spread of 129 feet and diameter at base of 4½ feet.
Reproduced from an Original Drawing by E. A. BURBANK.

The caption from the back of this photograph reads, "E.A. Burbank was a patient at Napa State Hospital at Imola but he was allowed to go out and sketch things that interested him in the area. A favorite subject was the firehouse then on Second Street Opposite Church Street. Other sketches can be seen at the Napa Firemen's Museum in Napa. This oak tree could be on the State Hospital Grounds." (Courtesy NCHS.)

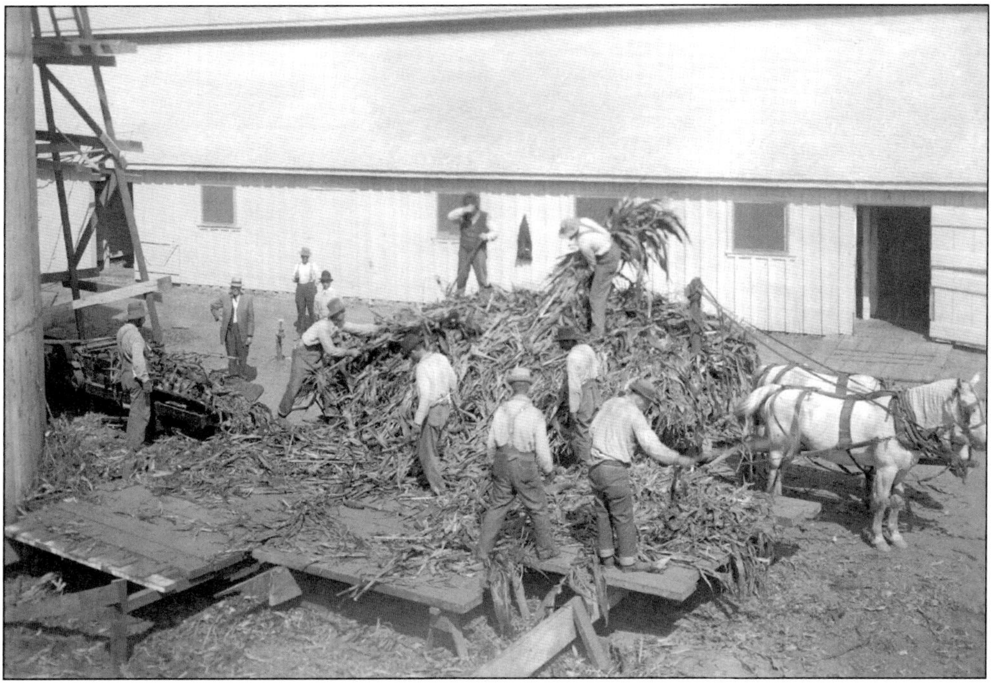

In 1920, the farm yielded 1,800 sacks of grain, 210 tons of hay, and 360 tons of cured hay, primarily used for the dairy operations. In 1923, workers and patients are seen filling the silo with hay grown on the hospital's farm that would be used as cattle feed. (Courtesy NSH.)

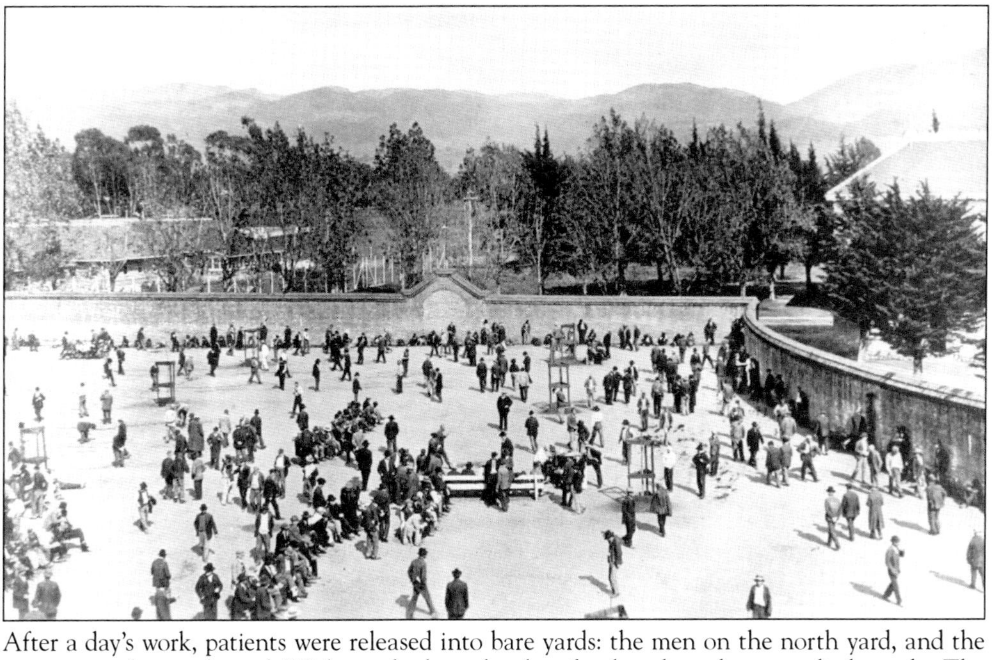

After a day's work, patients were released into bare yards: the men on the north yard, and the women on the south yard. With no shade and only a few benches, there was little to do. The buildings on the left behind the wall were Phillips Cottages, which were for working male patients who had grounds privileges. Those with either acute or chronic physical disease were moved to the infirmary and given 24-hour care. (Courtesy NCHS.)

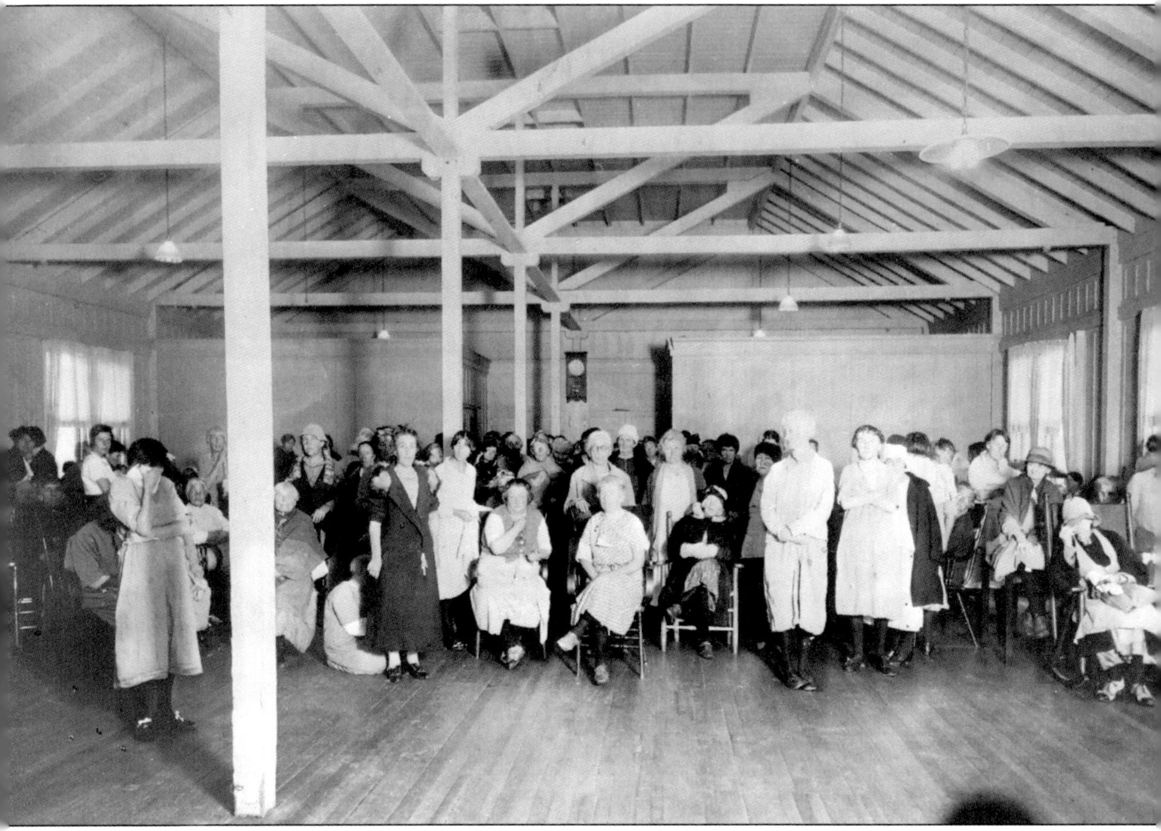

The superintendent's report stated that 386 patients were jammed into the notorious Dozier Cottage, pictured here in the mid-1930s. There were only a few chairs, and many patients had to stand or sit on the floor. Supt. T.H. Stice reported of conditions in the asylum: "The noise and confusion is bedlam." Crowding was commonplace in the Castle, where a typical ward had a capacity of 26 but housed 64 patients. (Courtesy NSH.)

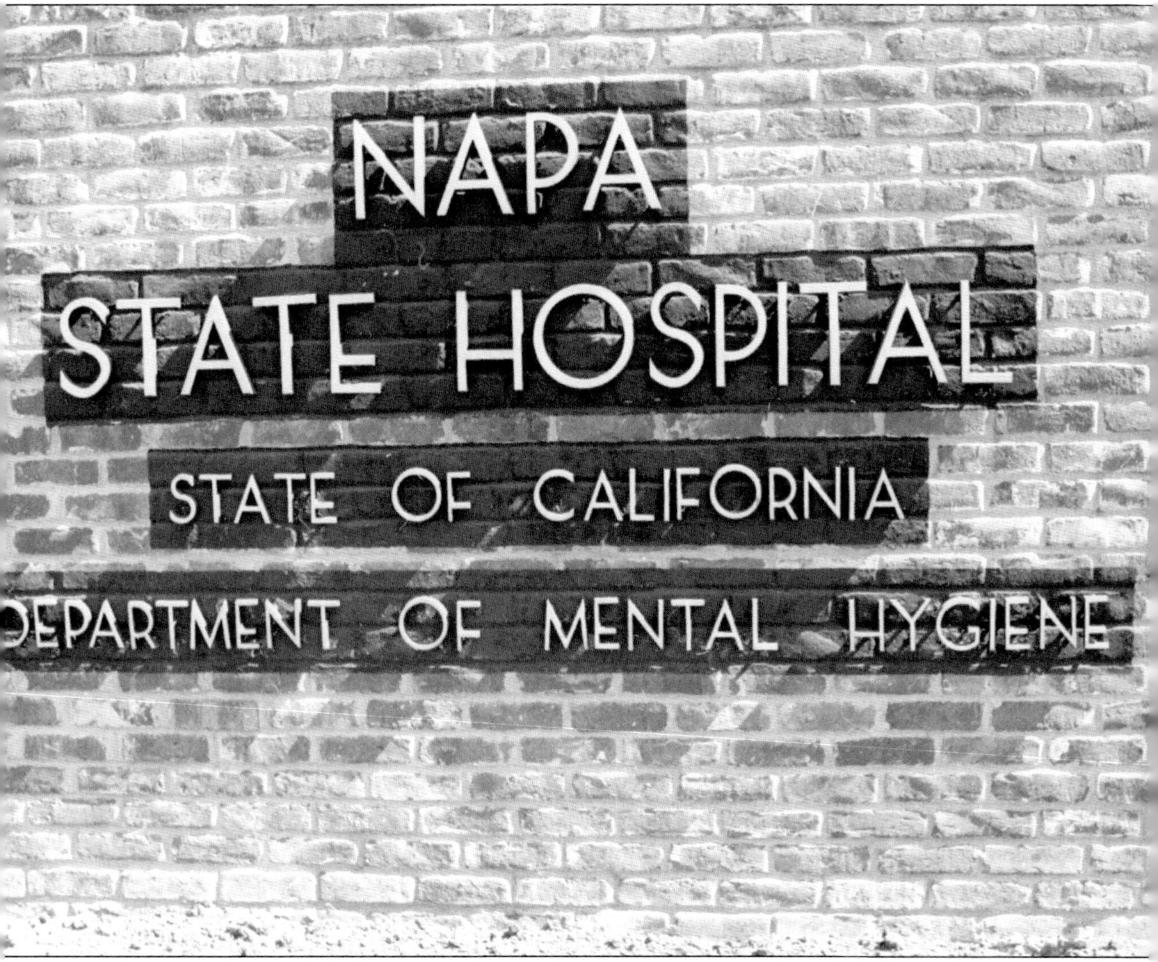

The Department of Institutions was created in Sacramento in 1922 to assume administration of state hospitals, reformatories, and homes for the blind. The Napa Asylum for the Insane changed its name to the Napa State Hospital in 1924, and "insanity" was thereafter referred to as "mental illness." In 1945, the Department of Institutions was renamed the Department of Mental Hygiene. (Courtesy NSH.)

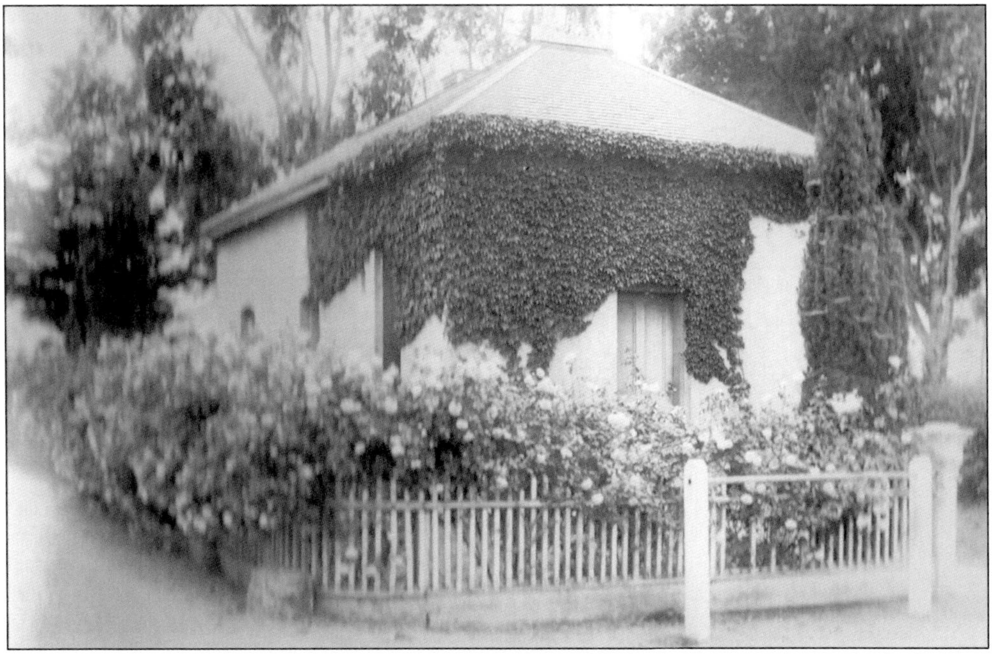

The hospital's morgue is pictured here in 1927. Unclaimed bodies were buried in unmarked graves in all of California's state hospitals. At Napa State Hospital, land that was later used for farm structures served as a "paupers' cemetery" until 1924. According to a *Napa Register* article, 4,363 adults are buried on the hospital grounds, while another 5,100 cremated remains of those who passed from 1924 to 1964 are located in a mass grave at the Chapel of the Chimes. The hospital has records of all those buried and cremated, but the exact location of the graves is unknown. (Courtesy CSA.)

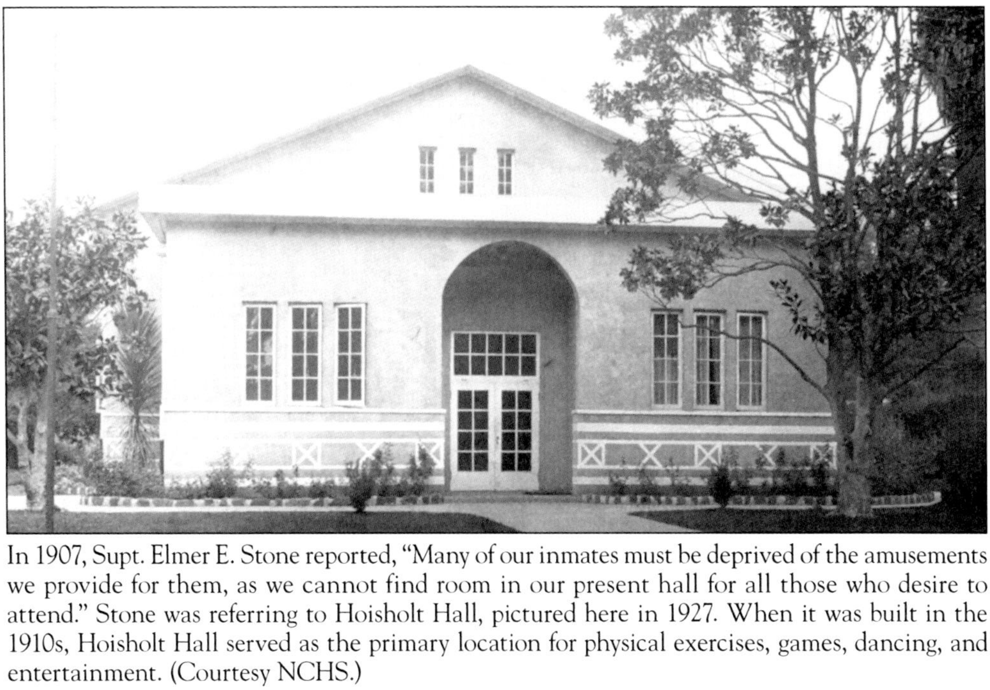

In 1907, Supt. Elmer E. Stone reported, "Many of our inmates must be deprived of the amusements we provide for them, as we cannot find room in our present hall for all those who desire to attend." Stone was referring to Hoisholt Hall, pictured here in 1927. When it was built in the 1910s, Hoisholt Hall served as the primary location for physical exercises, games, dancing, and entertainment. (Courtesy NCHS.)

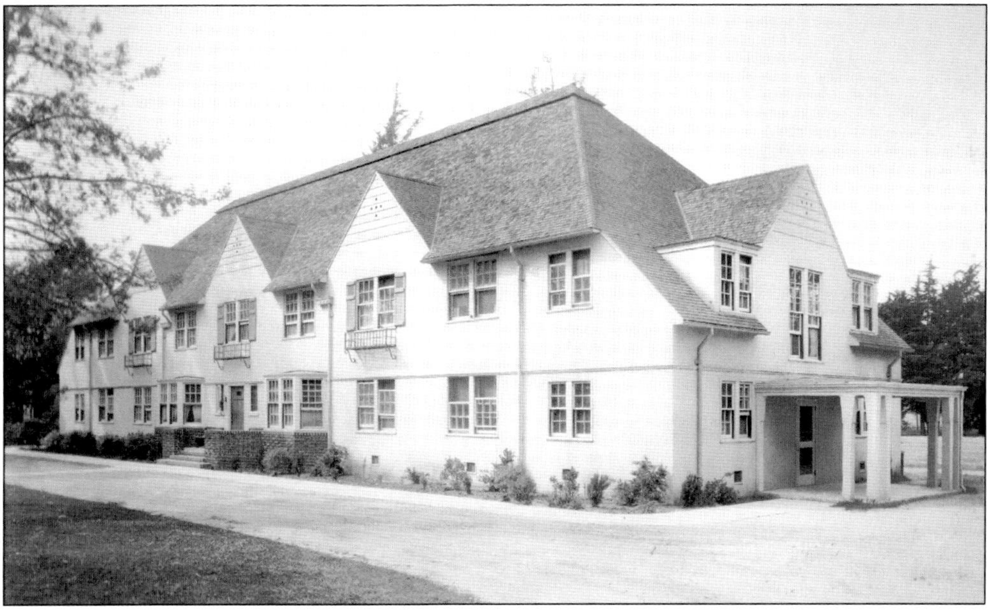

The married nurses' dorm was completed and opened in 1921, with room for 17 single women, five married couples who were both employees, and perhaps night attendants as well. The plans for this first employee dormitory included three dorms formed into a *U*-shaped complex with a north-facing courtyard, but the idea for a *U*-shaped layout was eventually dropped. (Courtesy CSA.)

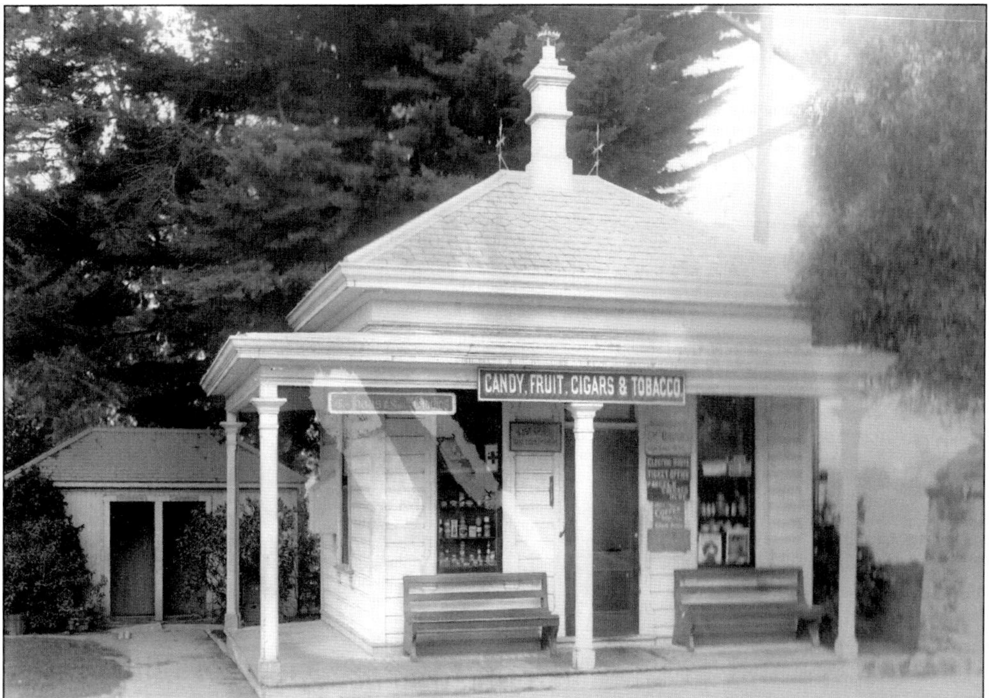

In the early part of the 20th century, souvenirs such as postcards of the hospital dairy herd and outlying buildings, as well as engraved spoons, were sold at the gift shop near the entrance, with proceeds going to hospital maintenance. (Courtesy CSA.)

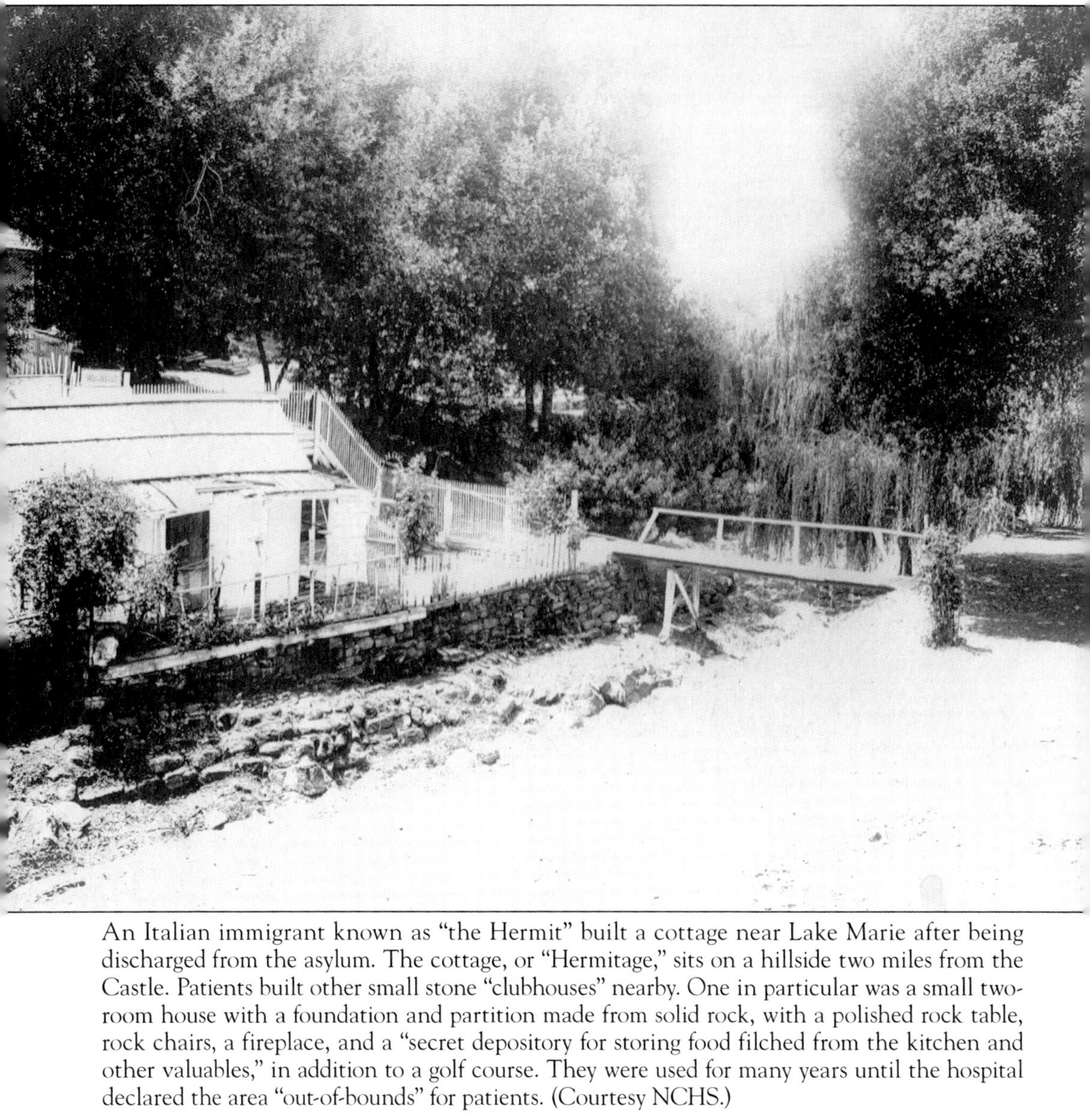

An Italian immigrant known as "the Hermit" built a cottage near Lake Marie after being discharged from the asylum. The cottage, or "Hermitage," sits on a hillside two miles from the Castle. Patients built other small stone "clubhouses" nearby. One in particular was a small two-room house with a foundation and partition made from solid rock, with a polished rock table, rock chairs, a fireplace, and a "secret depository for storing food filched from the kitchen and other valuables," in addition to a golf course. They were used for many years until the hospital declared the area "out-of-bounds" for patients. (Courtesy NCHS.)

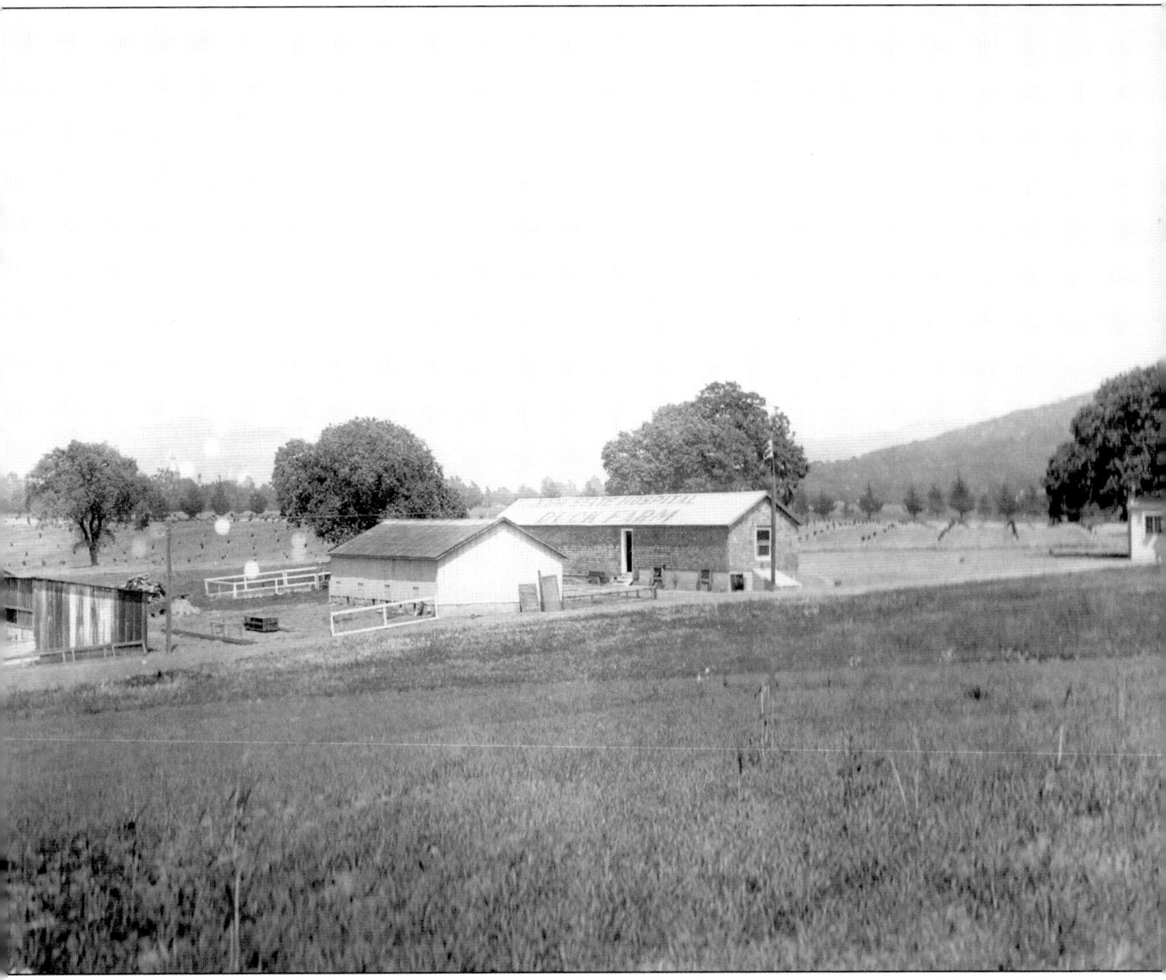

Pictured here in 1927 is the duck farm at Smith Brown Ranch, which is now part of Napa Valley College. Farming and poultry operations located there were critical to the survival of the institution, as was patient labor. Funds from the sale of products were used for building maintenance and the construction of new facilities for entertainment, treatment centers, and dormitories for nurses, which were built to ease overcrowding in the Castle. The duck farm was very successful and provided food for the Napa State Hospital as well as other institutions. The Napa State Hospital Ranch, used for cattle, was located east of Yountville. (Courtesy CSA.)

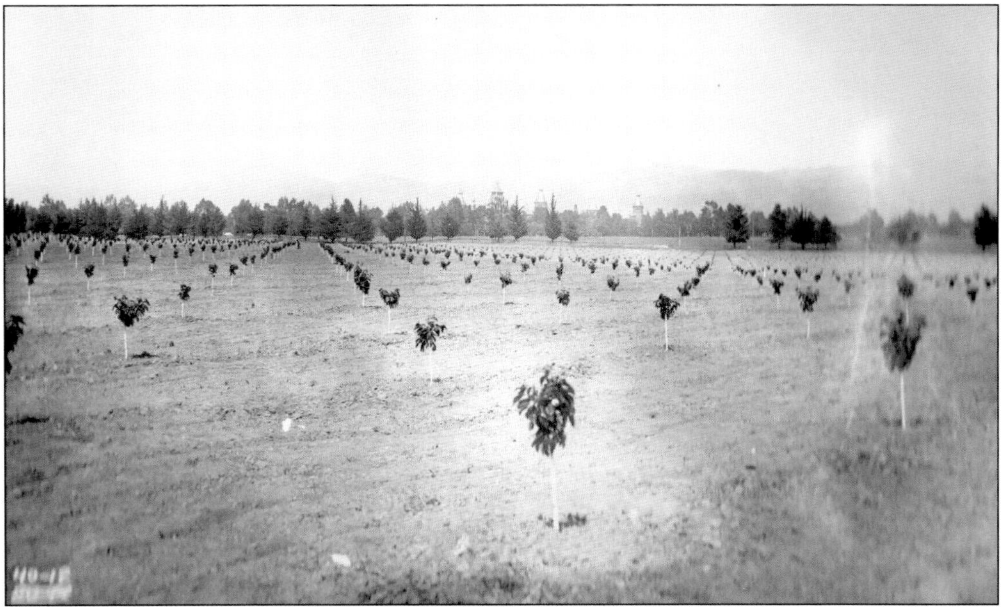

In this view of an orchard on the Smith Brown Ranch, the Castle is visible in the distance. (Courtesy CSA.)

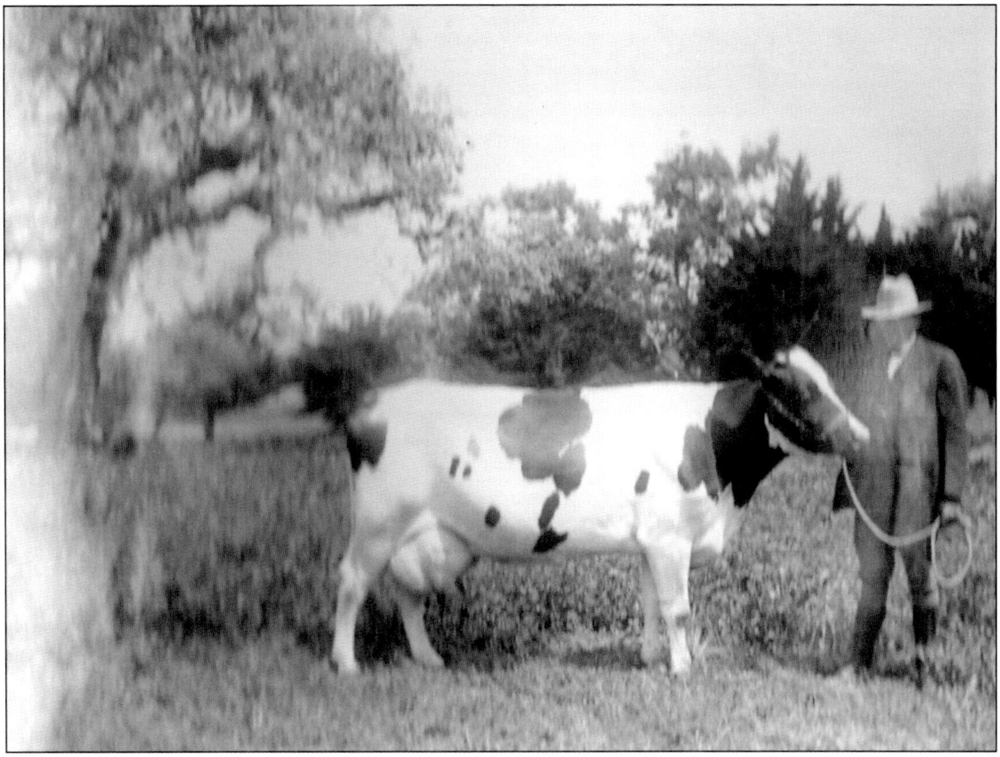

V.L. Heath, who managed the dairy department and whose efforts yielded high records for milk and butterfat content, is pictured here in 1927. The dairy department used the "utmost care in breeding and selection, using high record registered bulls and retaining only heifers from cows of high production." (Courtesy CSA.)

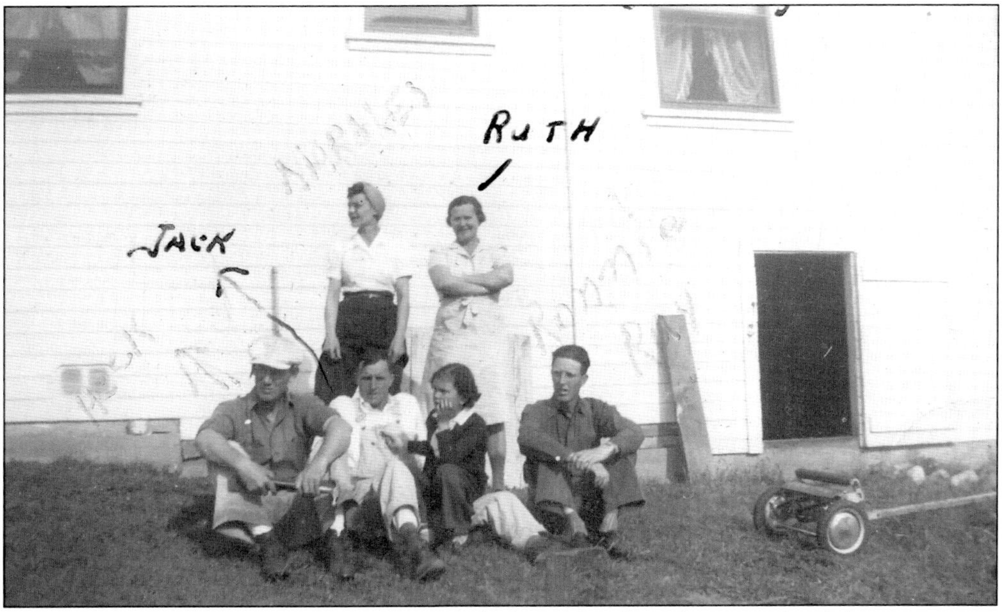

Three generations of the Nowlin family worked and lived on the grounds of the Napa State Hospital. Jack was a maintenance worker who, as an umpire for the City of Napa, organized many baseball games held on the hospital's baseball diamond. His wife, Ruth, was a psychiatric technician. Between Jack, his wife, his brother, his son, and his son's wife, the family provided over 100 years of service to the state. (Courtesy Cindi Hummer.)

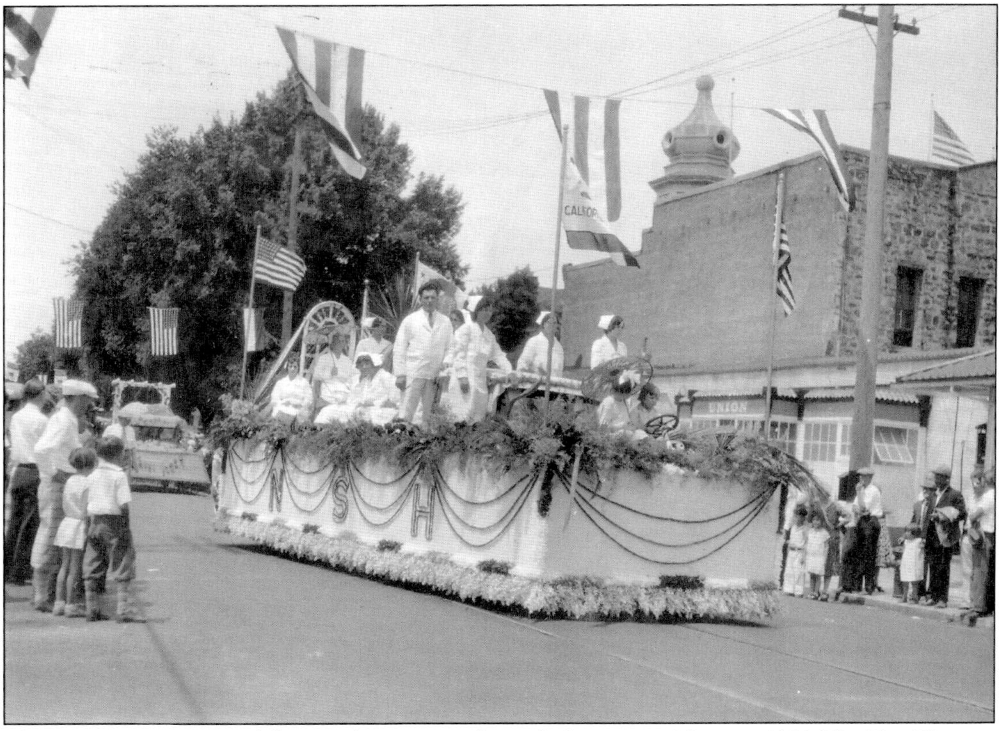

The Napa State Hospital float makes its way through downtown Napa in 1931. The Fox Theatre and *Napa Register* buildings are visible in the background. (Courtesy NCHS.)

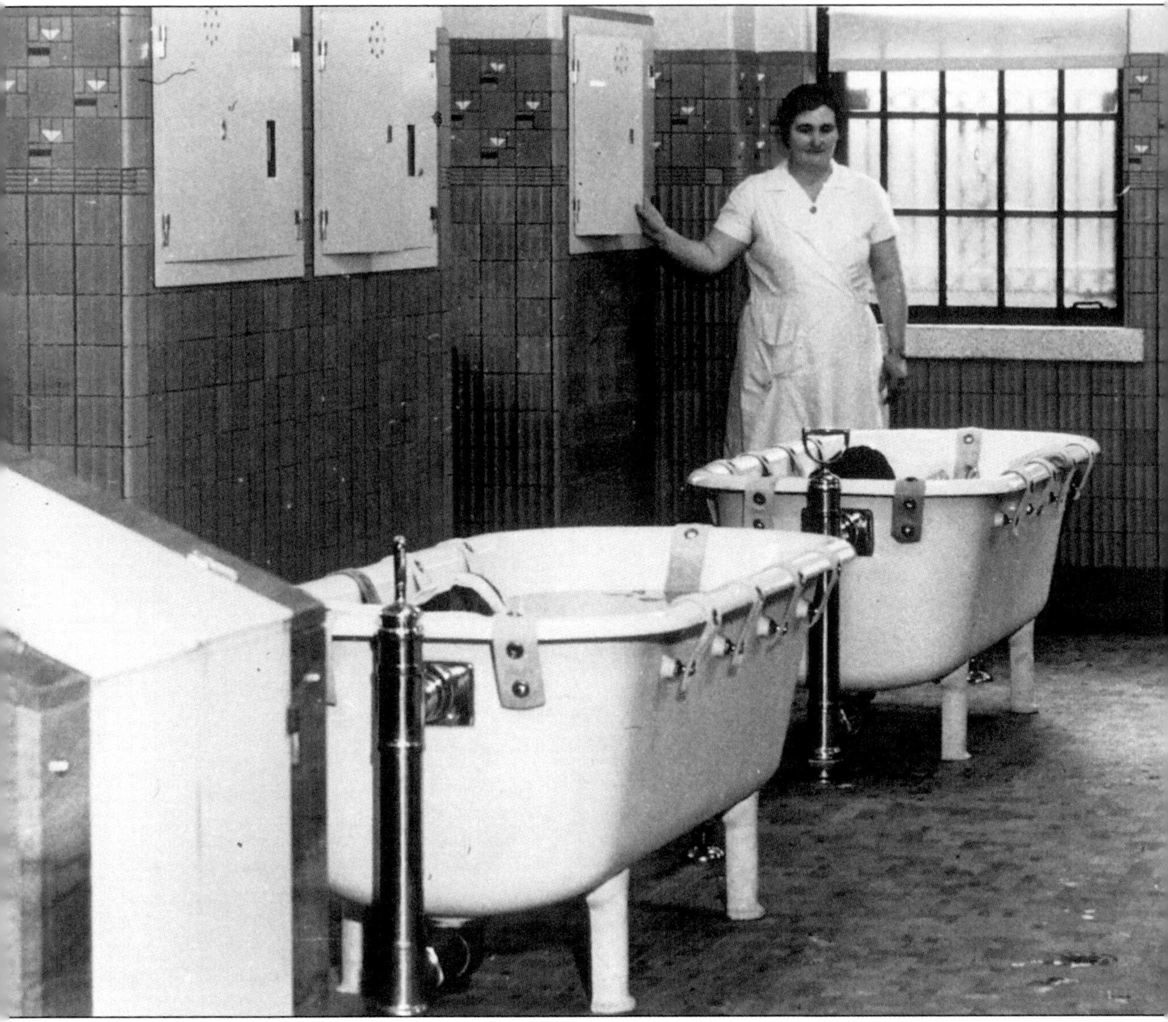

In the 1910s, hydrotherapy became standard practice in addition to mechanical restraints and drug therapy. A continuous bath, pictured here at the Pilgrim State Hospital in 1936, could last from hours to days and required around-the-clock attendants to drain and refill the tubs with water of varying temperatures. High-pressure sprays and hoses were also used to subdue patients, particularly veterans. Many physicians believed it relieved cerebral congestion, while others thought it helped to purge toxic impurities that led to insanity. (Courtesy Alfred Eisenstaedt, Pilgrim State Hospital.)

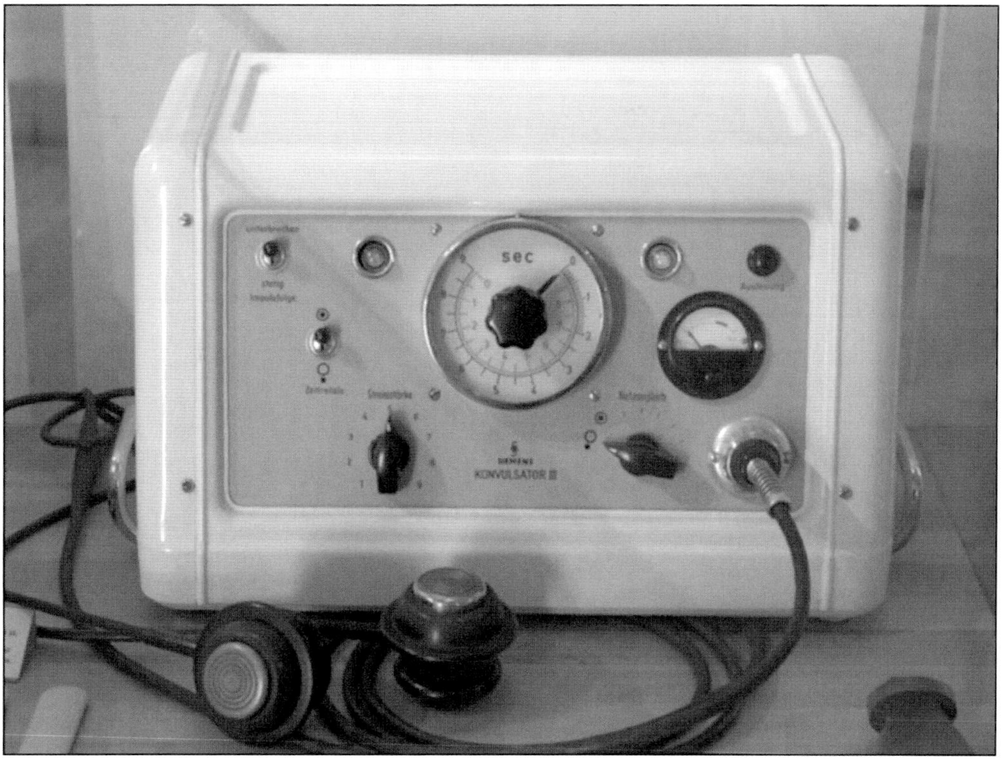

Treatments in the form of hydrotherapy, electroconvulsive therapy, leucotomy, sterilization, and clitoridectomy were performed in an attempt to subdue and permanently alter patients' behavior. The intent was to "cure" the patients as quickly as possible, ostensibly due to overcrowding in state hospitals. They were considered "approved scientific methods," and although they helped some people, there were numerous side effects and occasional deaths as a result of these treatments. Pictured here is an ECT machine, the Siemens Konvulsator III, which was commonly used around the country during this era.

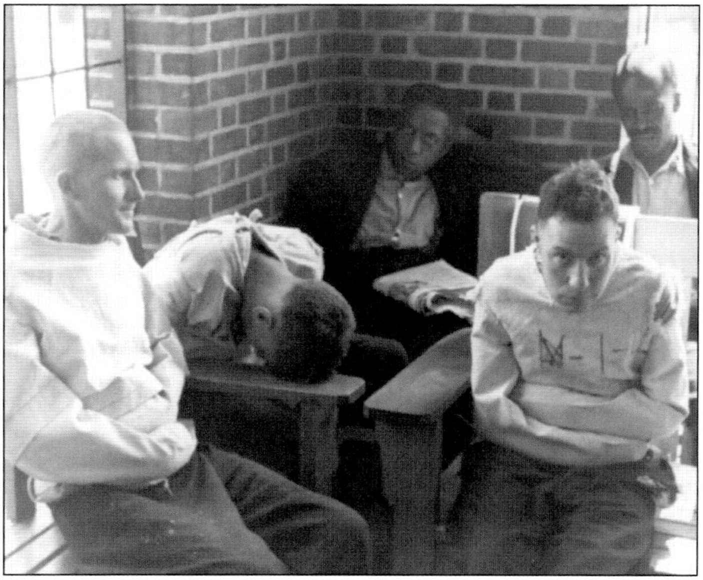

Unprovoked violence between patients and toward attendants in crowded wards was a part of daily life. Although many psychiatric facilities avoided the use of restraints, a violent patient was subdued with a straitjacket in some situations. Rendered vulnerable with the straitjacket, the restrained patient's peers had to be straitjacketed as well. (Courtesy Alfred Eisenstaedt, Pilgrim State Hospital.)

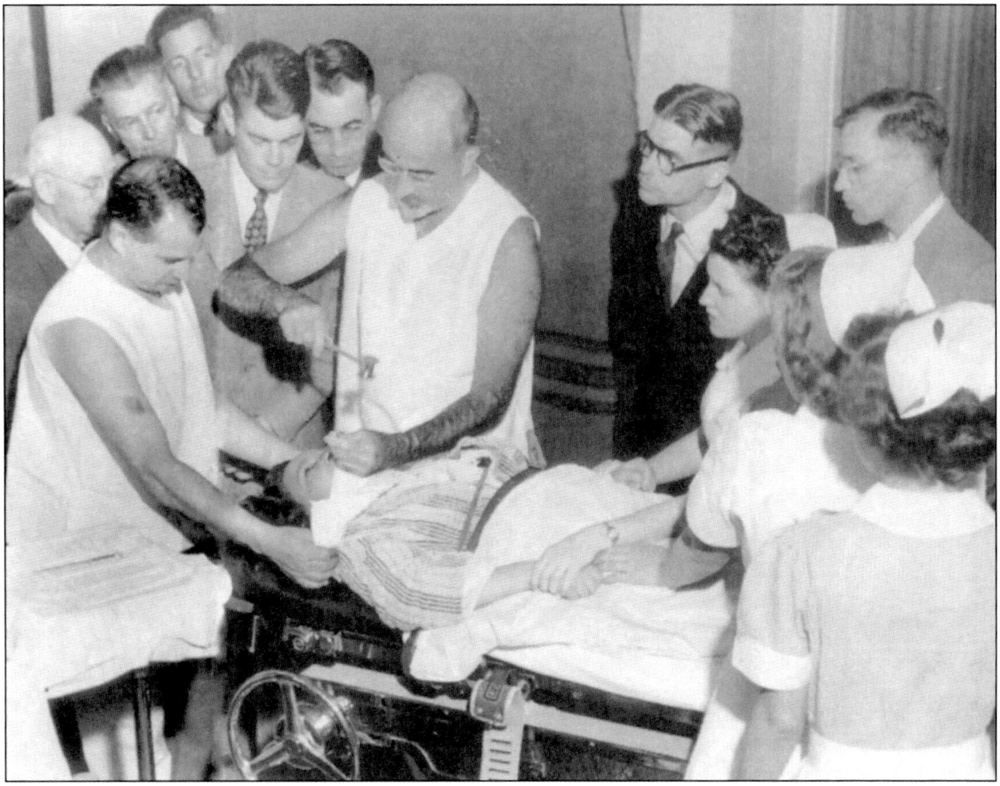

Despite major objections from the medical community when the procedure was first introduced, António Egas Moniz's leucotomy, or lobotomy, procedure eventually gained traction and was performed with alarming regularity in American hospitals in the 1940s and 1950s. In 1946, Walter Freeman simplified the procedure so that it could be performed in state hospitals with limited surgical facilities. It became known as transorbital, or "ice-pick," lobotomy, and by 1951 over 18,000 people had been lobotomized in the United States. Freeman spent some time at the Napa State Hospital and donated a collection of articles to the research library. (Courtesy CCHR International.)

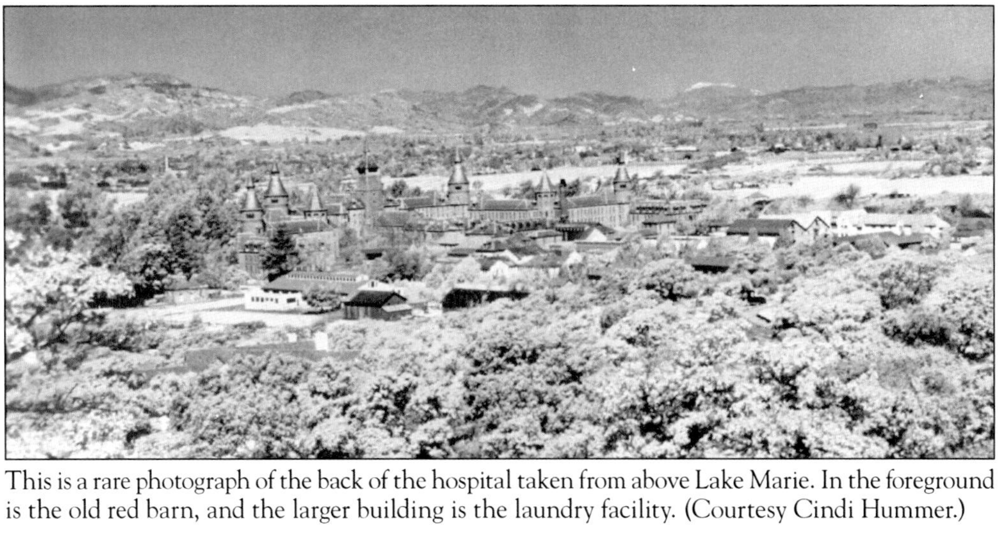

This is a rare photograph of the back of the hospital taken from above Lake Marie. In the foreground is the old red barn, and the larger building is the laundry facility. (Courtesy Cindi Hummer.)

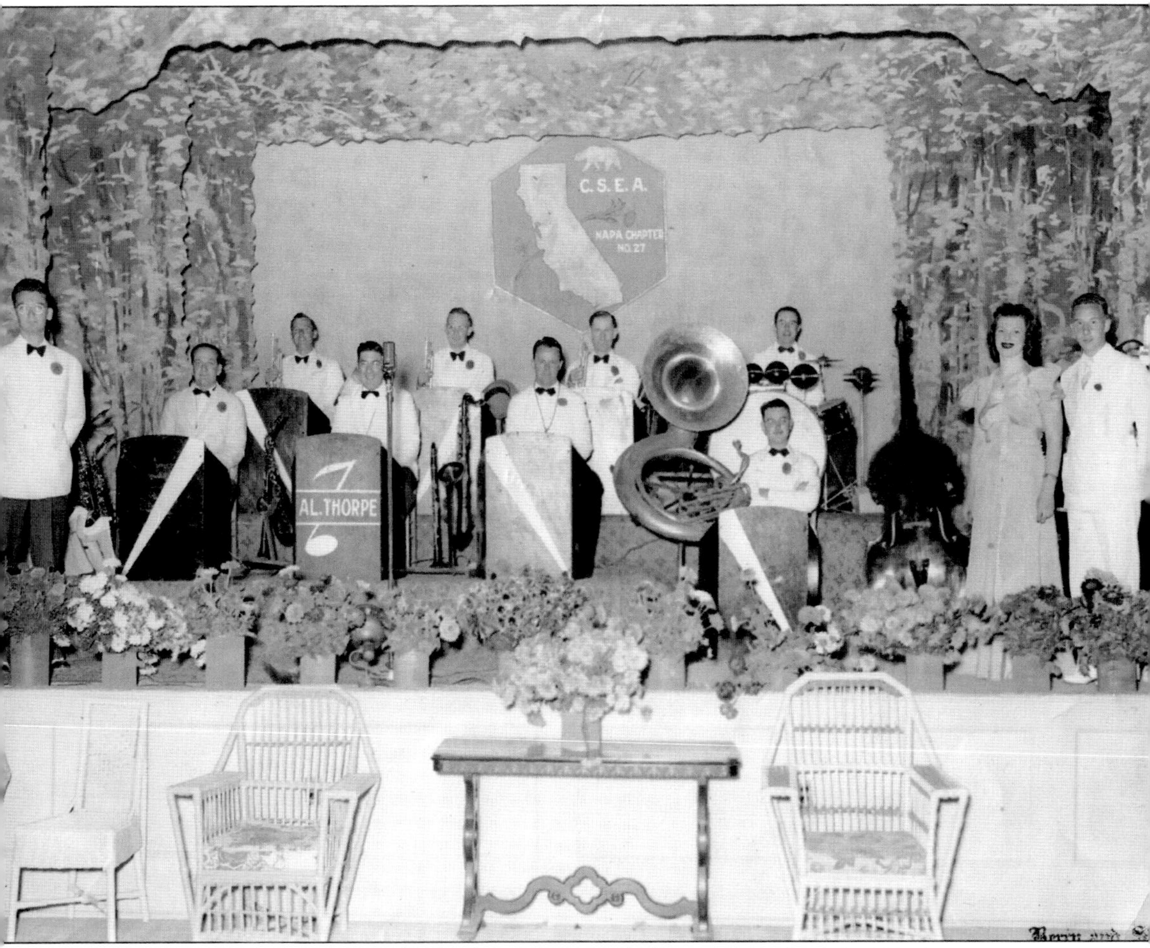

According to the caption on the back of this photograph dated September 15, 1938, the musicians are, from left to right, Al Thorpe, Dorman Jones, Hilary Helsley, Bob Walker, Eddie Zaro, Lowell Tate, "Chuck" Winter, Kenny Clark, Jack Cronhardt, "Jackie" Lytjen, and Jimmy Brown. The band performed regularly in Hoisholt Hall through the 1980s. (Courtesy NCHS.)

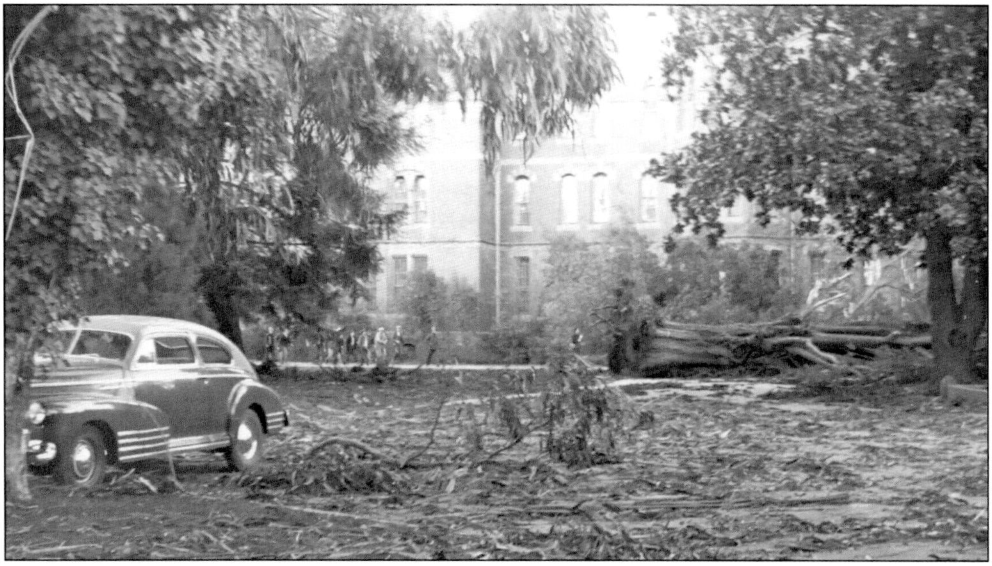

A severe windstorm inflicted damage in 1938. The grounds of the Napa State Hospital had 149 varieties of trees, which were an important aspect of the hospital's ability to provide treatment in a natural, serene environment. (Courtesy NSH.)

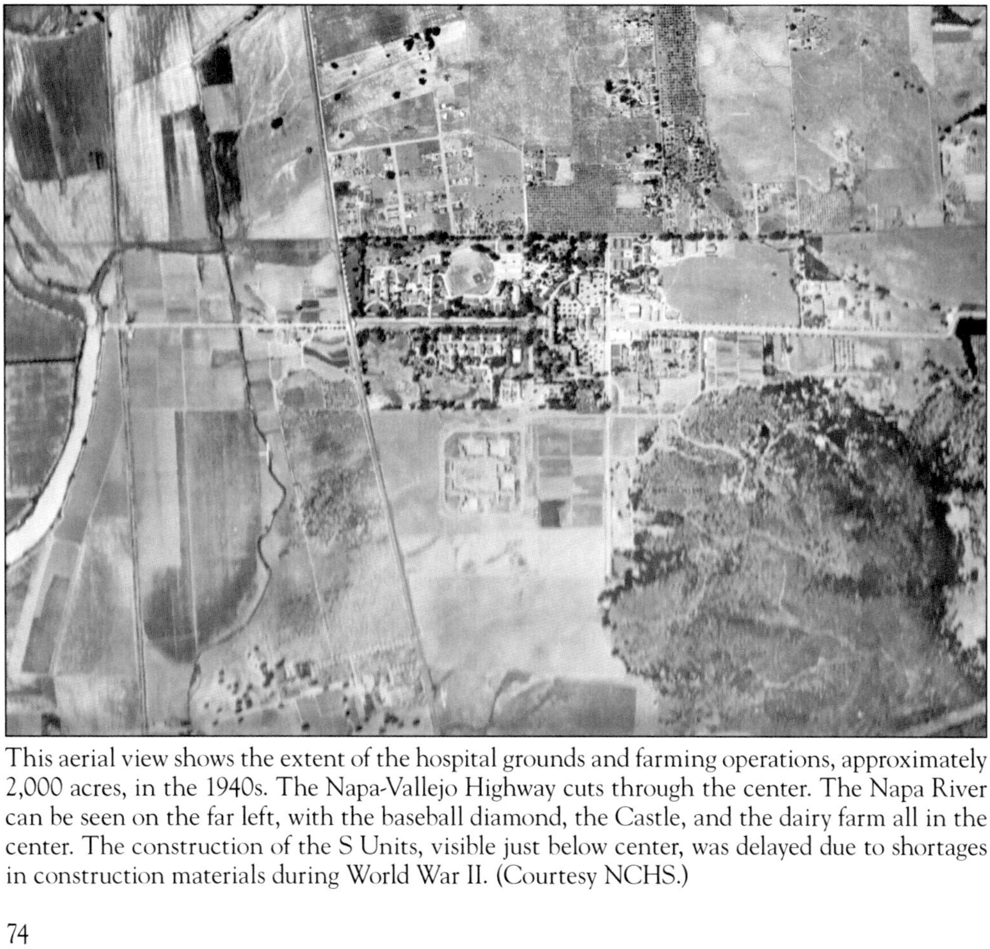

This aerial view shows the extent of the hospital grounds and farming operations, approximately 2,000 acres, in the 1940s. The Napa-Vallejo Highway cuts through the center. The Napa River can be seen on the far left, with the baseball diamond, the Castle, and the dairy farm all in the center. The construction of the S Units, visible just below center, was delayed due to shortages in construction materials during World War II. (Courtesy NCHS.)

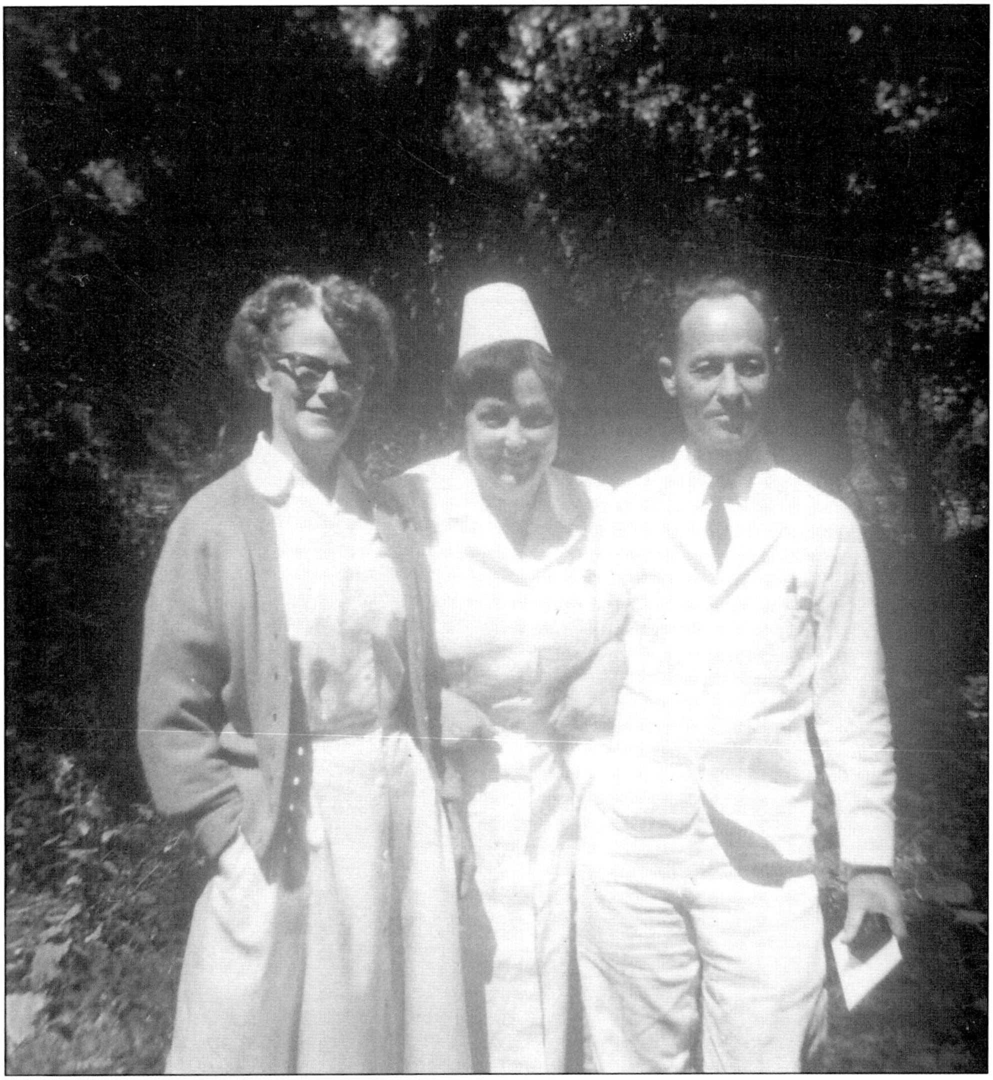

Psychiatric technicians are shown dressed in their starched whites in the 1940s. Former psychiatric attendant Jackie Hoyle recalled in a 2007 *Napa Marketplace* article that she had to buy her uniform from the local Albertson's Department Store, and it was made of "fabric like cardboard." She added, "I had fun and a lot of friends. People worked very hard and were good to the patients." During this time, ward psychiatric technicians bathed patients, accompanied them to the dining room, and walked them out to the yard in the afternoon. They were required to have three months of training and pass a test prior to working on the wards. (Courtesy Cindi Hummer.)

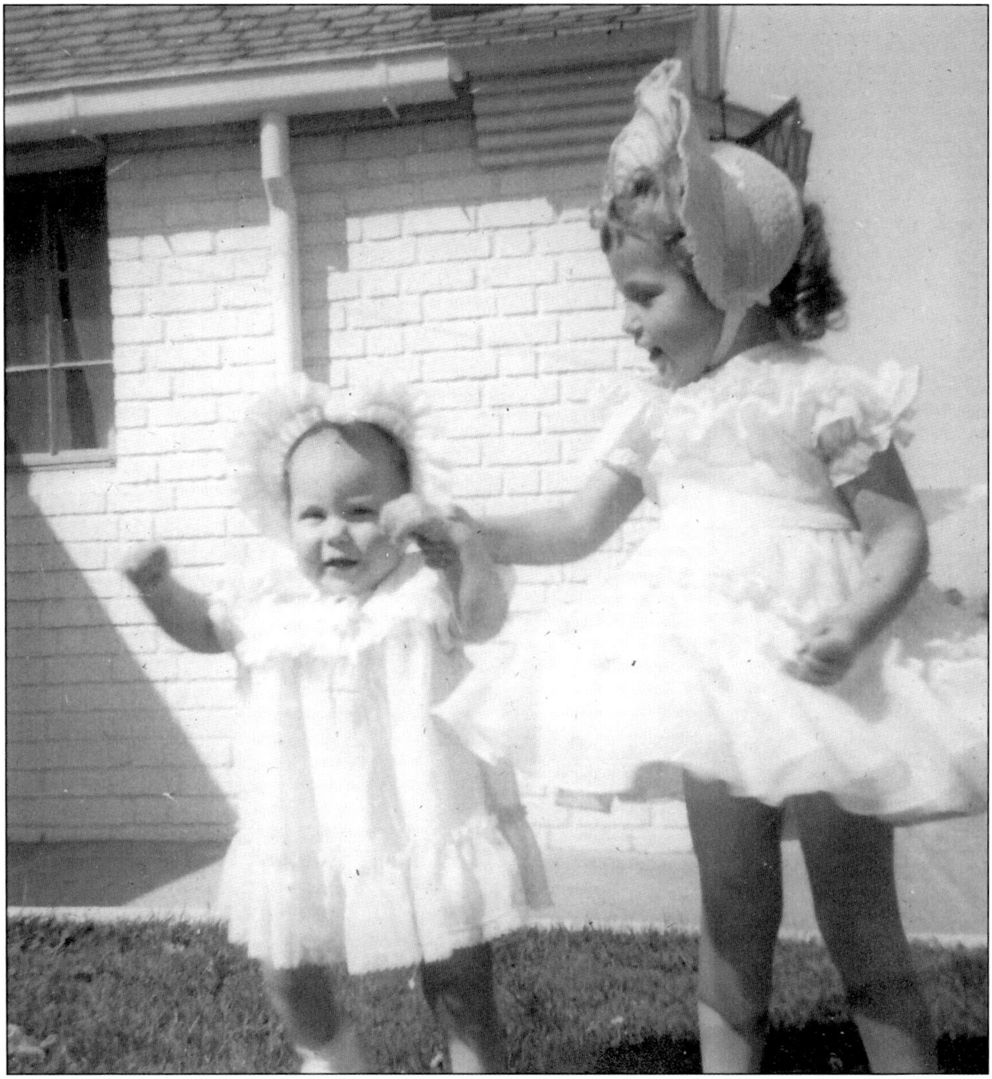

In this image are Cindi Hummer (left) and her sister on the grounds of Napa State Hospital. She recalls a "close-knit community" where she spent her childhood playing on a giant swing set located near the hospital entrance and picking cherries from the orchard across the highway. She and her sister, determined to "set them free," once released prized steers from the hospital dairy. The firefighters, one of whom was her father, were called in to retrieve the roaming herd. (Courtesy Cindi Hummer.)

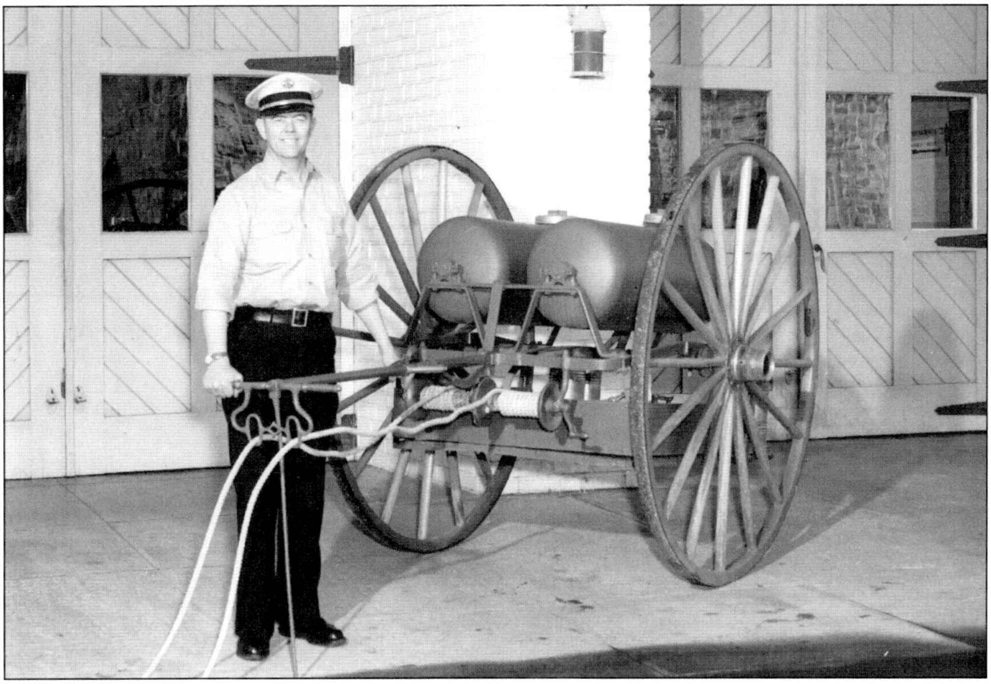

Napa State Hospital firefighters, known as the bucket brigade and established in 1875, were an integral part of the institution. In 1882, when fire extinguishers, hydrants, and hoses were installed to replace buckets, the Asylum Hose Company was assembled. It was primarily made up of ward attendants. (Courtesy NCHS.)

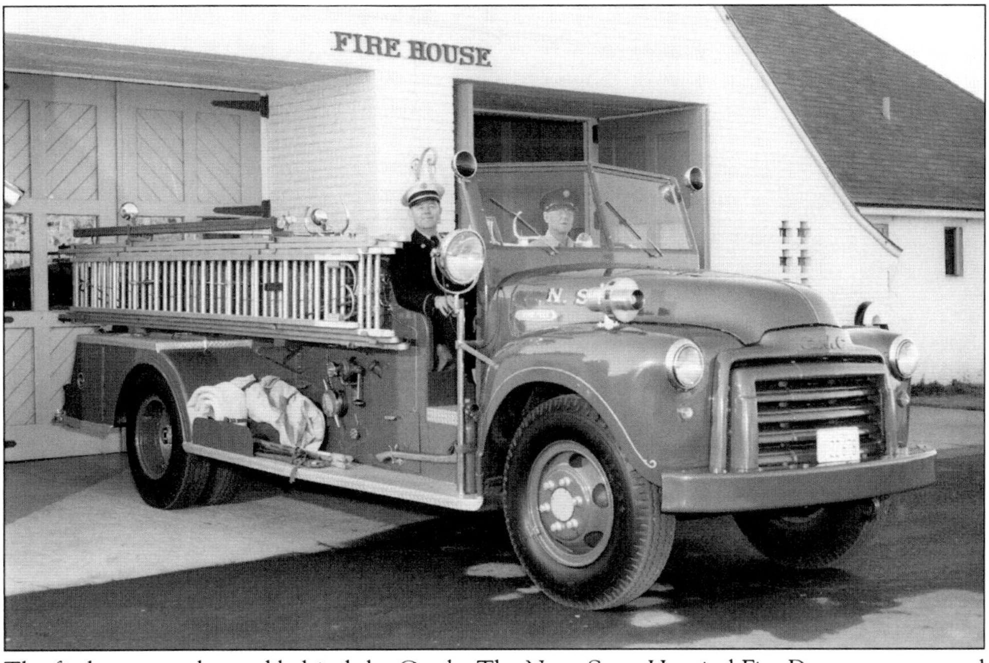

The firehouse was located behind the Castle. The Napa State Hospital Fire Department served as backup for psychiatric technicians when fights broke out between patients in the wards. They were also called in for emergencies all over Napa County as needed. (Courtesy NCHS.)

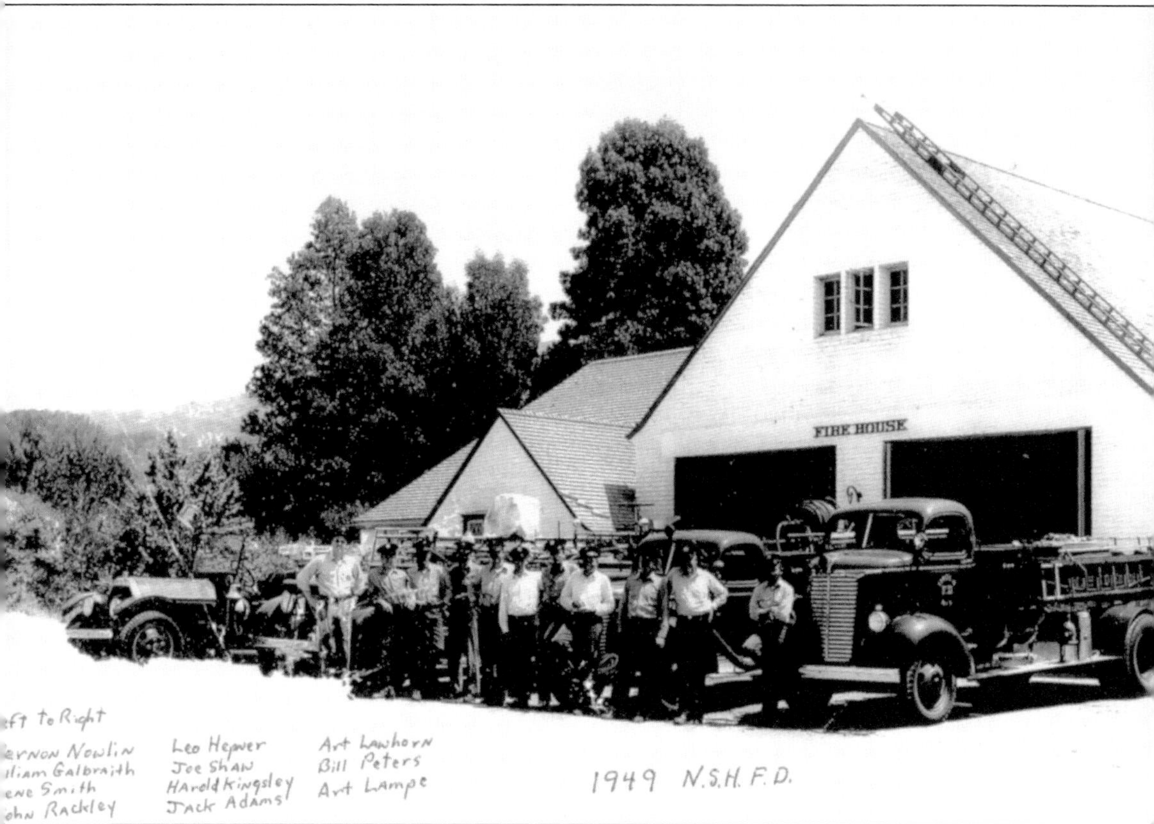

The Napa State Hospital Fire Department staff of 1949 included, from left to right, Vernon Nowlin, William Galbraith, Gene Smith, John Rackley, Leo Hepner, Joe Shaw, Harold Kingsley, Jack Adams, Art Lanhorn, Bill Peters, and Art Lampe. Darrell Turner, whose parents both retired from Napa State Hospital, recalls an idyllic childhood spent playing on the grounds and fishing by the farm ward with other employees' children. Firefighters lived in the firehouse, and Darrell fondly recollects visiting his father and the sense of extended family and community. Darrell also worked at Napa State Hospital, first assisting psychiatric technicians in the children's ward and later becoming a psychiatric technician himself, as well as a part-time firefighter. (Courtesy Darrell Turner.)

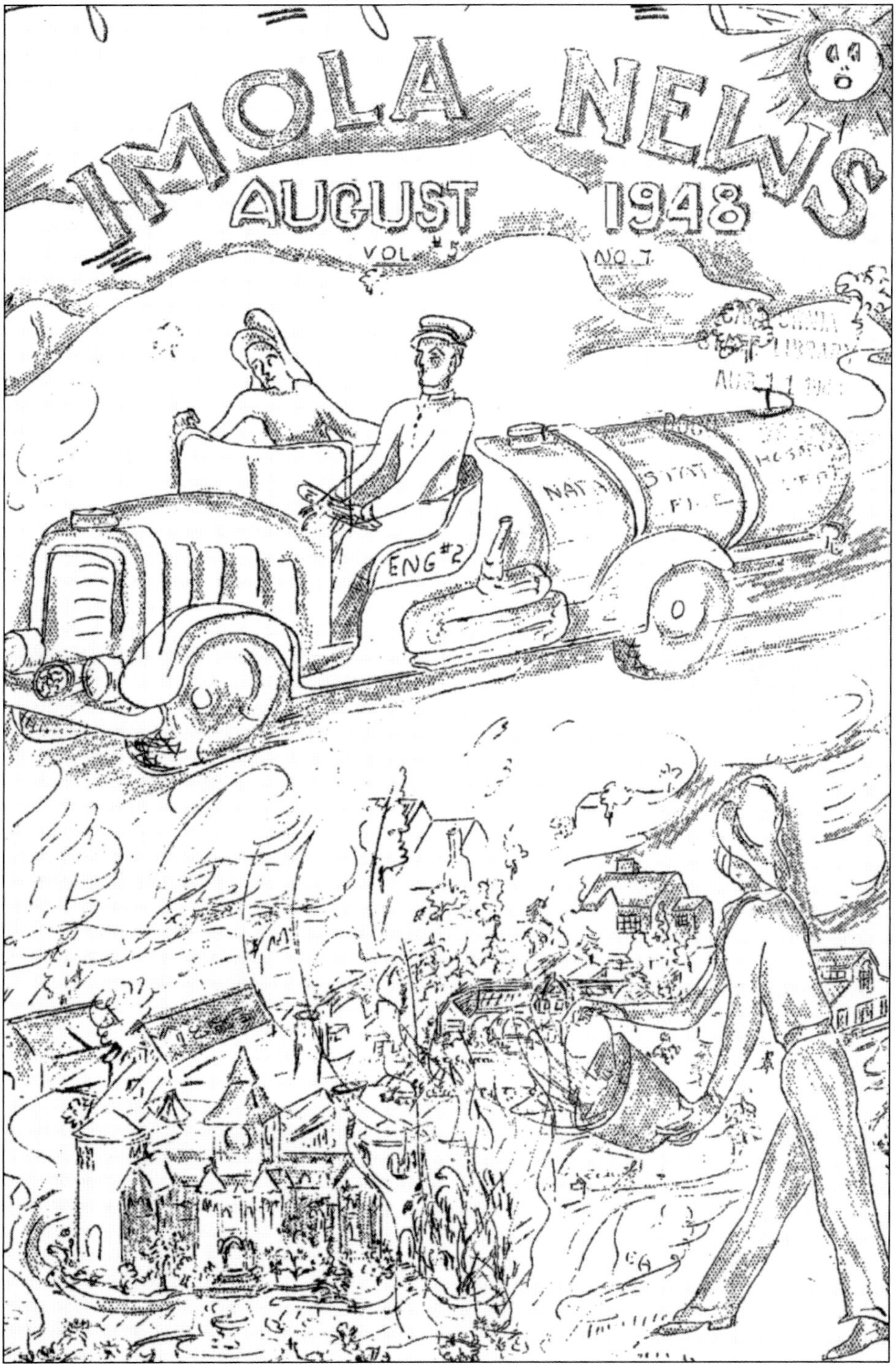

The Napa State Hospital firefighters were featured on the cover of this patient-run newsletter in 1948. Inside is an article recounting a hike and picnic to Lake Marie, where patients discovered, among other things, the remnants of an old stone cottage built by patients as well as stone fences constructed when the land was part of a rancho. (Courtesy Larry Seaton.)

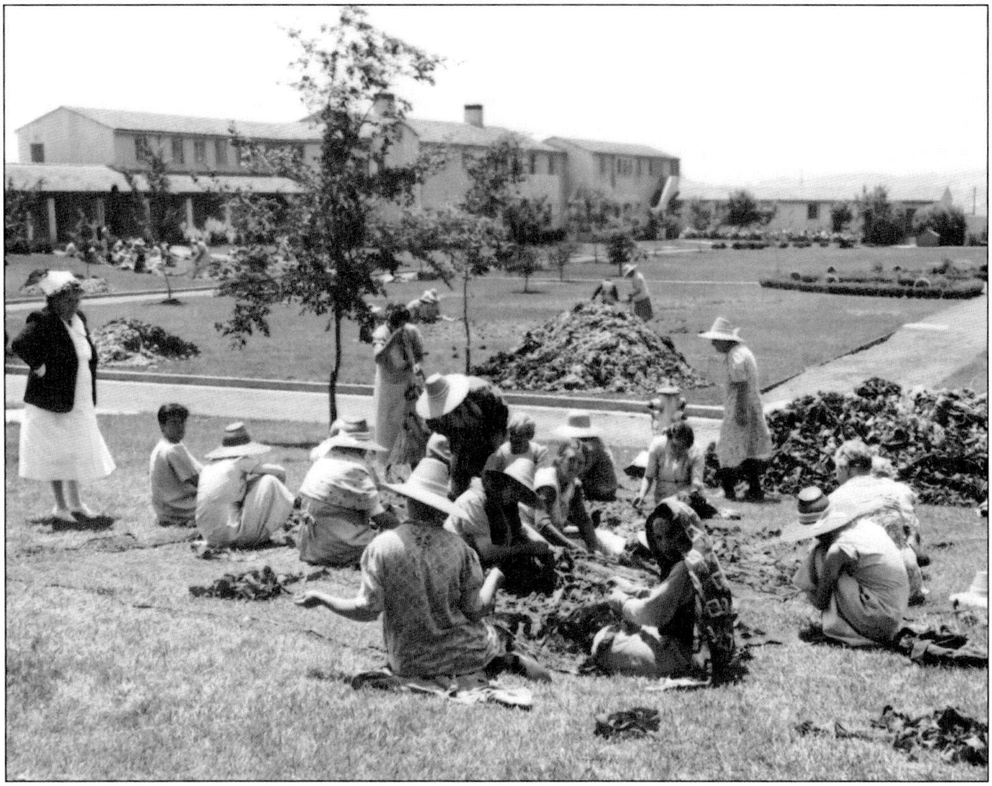

Patients in the S Unit courtyard are working on a World War II project making camouflage netting, one of the many ways in which the institution assisted the war effort. (Courtesy NSH.)

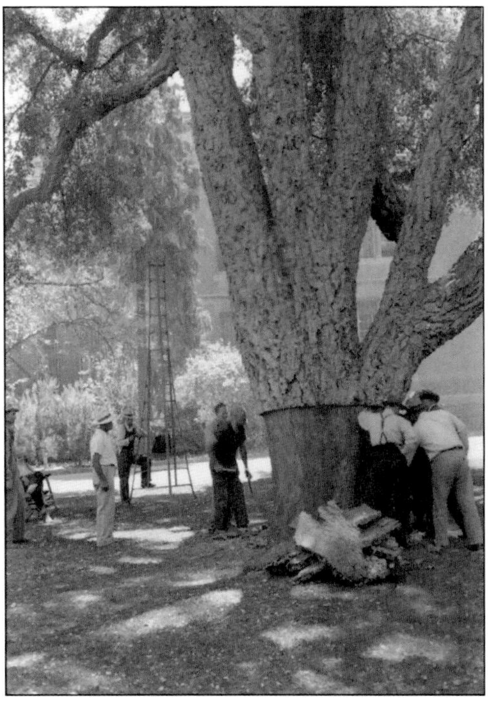

During World War II, the Navy used the newly built Q Ward as a hospital facility called the Mare Island Naval Hospital annex. At the time, cork was used for industrial applications such as insulation, and, as shown here, the U.S. Navy debarked some of the cork trees on the Napa State Hospital grounds. The cork was unusable, but the event provided a great public relations opportunity for Napa State Hospital. (Courtesy Fritz-Metcalf Photograph Collection.)

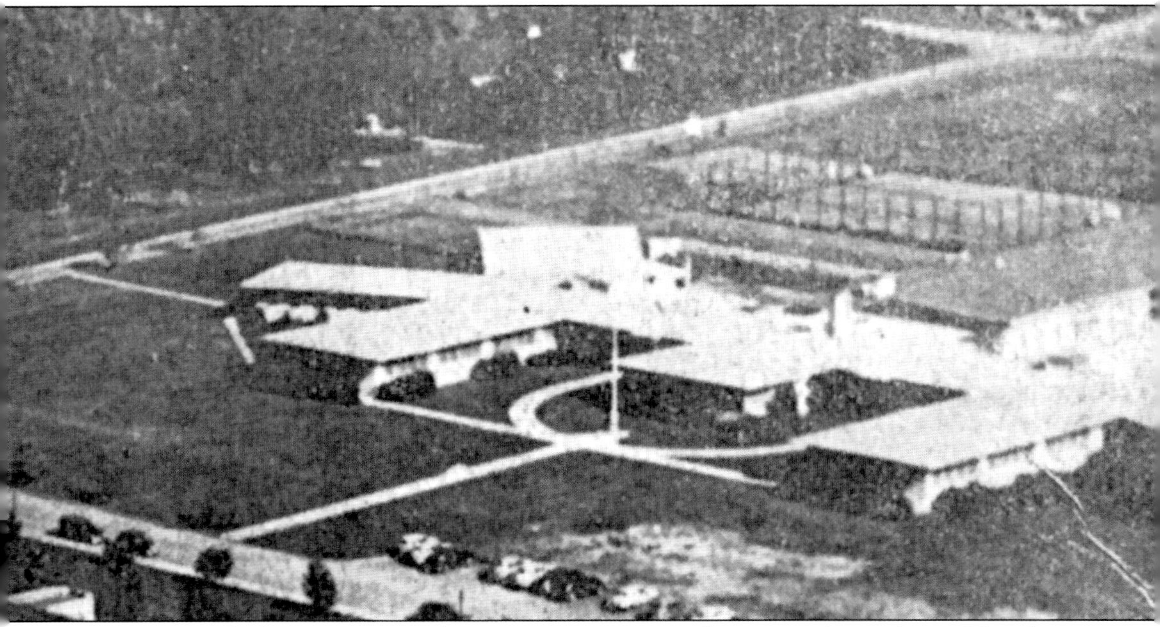

In Jack Reynolds's letters written to the Napa County Historical Society in September and October of 1998, according to a former Navy corpsman who lived there in 1944–1945, corpsmen lived in temporary barracks built in 1917 at the intersection of Cedar and Madrone Avenues. They enjoyed swimming in Lake Camilla, eating apricots from a nearby orchard, and either walking or taking taxis into downtown Napa for a night out. They also often played pool with the attendants in the Castle, which he called "spooky as hell" and "eery [sic] at night." The Q Unit was returned to the hospital in 1946. (Courtesy NCHS.)

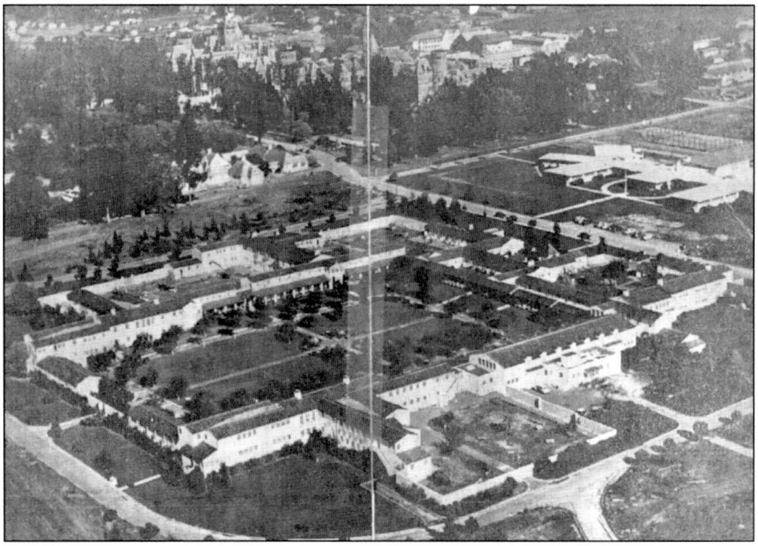

This 1940s aerial view shows the completed S Units in the center and the Q Units in the upper right. The Q Ward was built for tuberculosis patients, but by the time it was completed, better treatments meant it was no longer needed for that purpose. (Courtesy NCHS.)

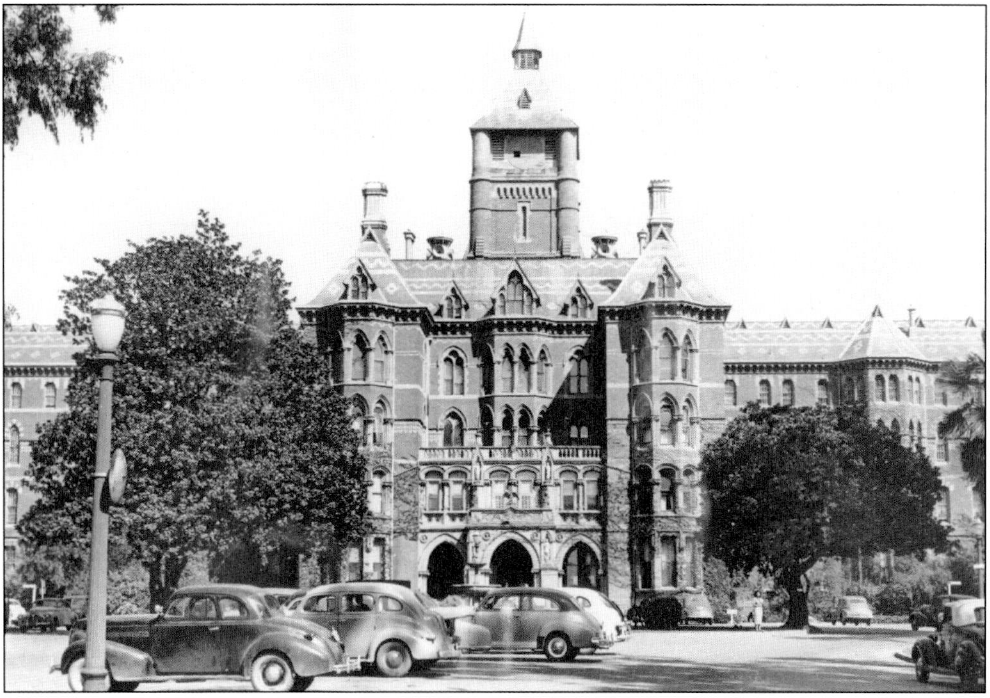

Complaints of overcrowding in California's state hospitals and reports of hazardous conditions from the fire marshal led Gov. Earl Warren to tour of all of the state institutions in 1942. He declared Napa State Hospital a "firetrap." In another survey, Dora Shaw Heffner, state director of institutions, confirmed the reports, and she recommended bedridden patients be immediately transferred to temporary quarters. (Courtesy NCHS.)

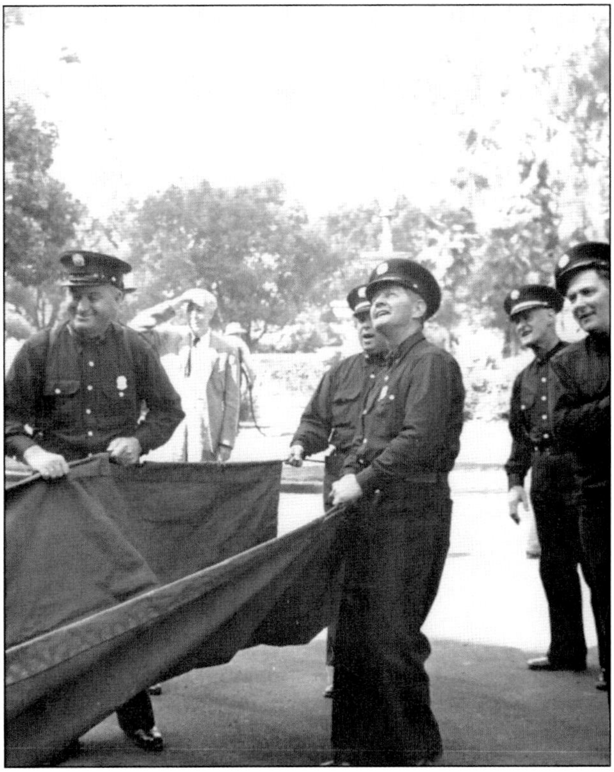

An escape canvas chute, shown here during a drill, was used to evacuate bedridden patients from the Castle. The 1943 evacuation was a direct result of a shortage of staff due to military service and unsafe conditions. The only means of egress in and out of the Castle were steep, unlighted spiral stone stairways in each of the seven towers. (At right, courtesy NCHS; below, Cindi Hummer.)

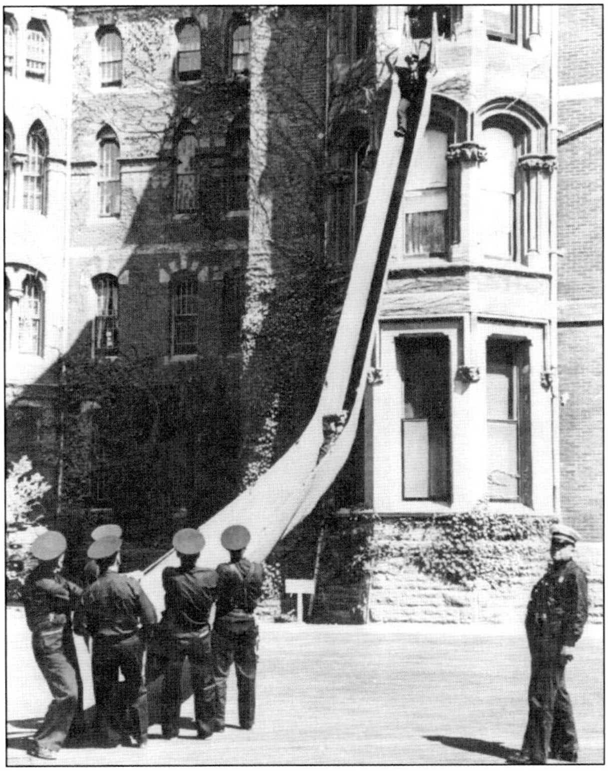

"Give Light and the People Will Find Their Own Way."

The San Francisco News

A Scripps-Howard Newspaper

presents a
reprint of

People in the Dark

A Series of Articles on California's Hospital System for the Mentally Sick

Written by Al Ostrow—Photographs by Robert J. Warren

A SUMMARY

To provide the public and Legislature with a possible guide to constructive improvement of California's care of its mentally ill, The News sent Reporter Al Ostrow and Photographer Robert J. Warren on a 2000-mile tour. They made a complete inspection of each state mental hospital in the most thorough informal investigation of this type ever attempted. They set up a problem of tremendous importance, which the people of California must solve.

Here is a summary of their findings, as disclosed in a series of articles entitled "People in the Dark":

OVERCROWDING.—About 7000 more patients than their "rated capacity" are jammed into the state hospitals. As a result, beds are packed into wards only a few inches apart, and many patients sleep in [illegible] hallways and on the floor. Dining rooms cannot accommodate the crowd, and eating conditions are often unpleasant.

TREATMENT.—Most state hospitals were designed chiefly as housing units, and have few facilities for treating patients. Even with such facilities as are available, the small but competent staffs are inadequate to give all patients the amount of personal attention required to assure maximum improvement. As a result, thousands of patients sit around and deteriorate. Their support becomes a permanent charge against the state.

EXPENSES.—The state spends only a little more than a dollar a day for each mental hospital patient, as contrasted with expenditures of $5 to $10 a day for the physically ill in general hospitals—this in spite of medical opinion that ailments of the mind require greater care and attention if cures are to be effected.

BUILDINGS.—Many state hospital buildings are antiquated, long condemned firetraps. Mental patients can recover more quickly in pleasant surroundings, but the atmosphere of most mental hospitals is drab and unpleasant.

THE AGED.—Thousands of senile old people sit about the hospitals in rags and tatters because the state has been unable to purchase proper clothing for them. Little or no treatment is provided for them.

ALCOHOLICS.—Alcoholic patients are also sent to mental hospitals, where the program for them is very limited. Some public health authorities advocate establishment of separate institutions for care of alcoholism.

COMMITMENT LAW.—Psychiatrists consider California's commitment law, which requires legal hearings and the making of a court record before most patients can be admitted to a mental hospital, to be [illegible]. They want the law changed to permit two doctors to commit a patient without court action if relatives agree. On the other hand, some judges believe such an amendment might deprive citizens of their freedom without "due process of law," since most patients are kept behind locked doors at a mental hospital and many may be there for life. This conflict must be resolved if all who need care are to have it.

PREVENTION.—The recently established Langley Porter Clinic has proved that much mental illness may be checked in early stages, before a patient requires hospitalization. California's mental health program is inadequate. Clinic facilities are not available in most parts of the state, thus providing no "out patient" care for patients discharged from the hospitals, but who need further help for complete recovery.

RESEARCH.—Research should be a major function of a mental hospital, being the only hope for many otherwise "hopeless" cases. State hospitals are conducting no research projects of any consequence.

NEGLECT.—The state hospitals have been neglected for decades. Legislators have been more concerned with political matters, so hospital appropriations have been ruthlessly trimmed.

PROGRAM.—Governor Earl Warren, who calls these conditions "a shame to the State of California," has made vigorous efforts to correct the situation. He obtained a 17-million-dollar appropriation from the Legislature for new buildings, beating down powerful opposition of interests wanting to earmark the funds for more political purposes. However, the building program has been blocked by the sharp rise in construction costs. Another 28 million dollars will be needed if the projects are to be completed. More money is needed to provide larger staffs, nursing, and other facilities.

FUTURE.—Only enlightened public interest in the welfare of the mentally ill can insure improvement of deplorable conditions in the state hospitals and overcome the general disinterest of politicians in the subject.

IMPORTANCE.—Mental illness is steadily increasing. Like physical disease, it may affect any one. Being mentally sick should carry no more stigma than physical illness. The U. S. Public Health Service estimates that one out of every 20 Americans will spend part of his life in a mental hospital. Therefore, conditions in mental hospitals are a vital concern to every one.

PRIVATE SANITARIUMS.—Officials of the State Department of Mental Hygiene declare that private institutions which permitted admittedly objectional features found in state hospitals would be promptly closed. Private sanitariums charge such high fees that most mentally ill persons who require hospitalization must be sent to the state institutions, where many are treated free and the families of others are charged up to $40 a month for their care. There are many charity patients.

An Example of Public Service in Journalism

In 1947, the *San Francisco News* published a lengthy exposé on the "deplorable" conditions found in California state hospitals. Its aim was to shed light on hospital inmates who were living in severely overcrowded institutions and in a shroud of darkness. The title also referred to the general public, whose ignorance made them "people in the dark" about the realities facing the mentally ill who could not afford treatment in private psychiatric hospitals. The public responded favorably to the article, which has been attributed to shifting attention back to the level of care in state hospitals. (Courtesy NSH.)

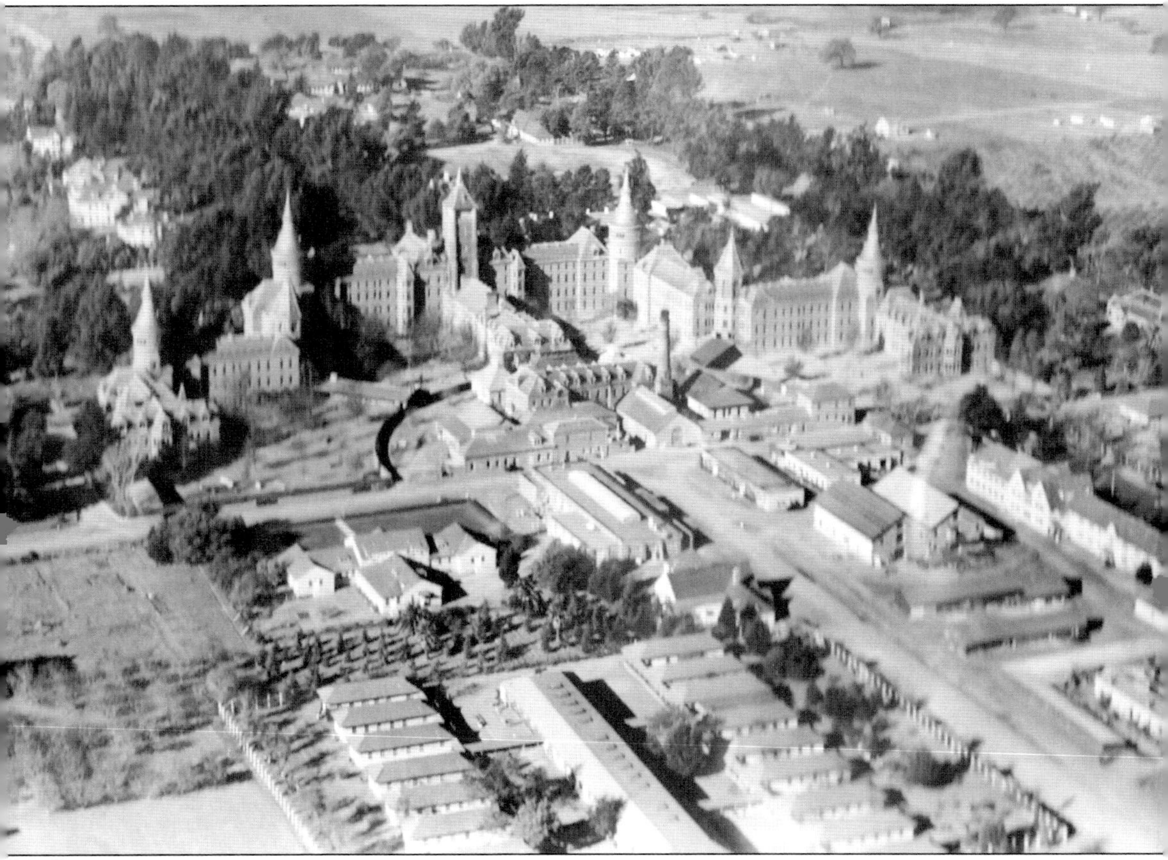

Changes in treatment for the mentally ill required modern treatment and surgery centers. In 1942, state fire marshal Joe R. Yockers notified Gov. Earl Warren of the buildings' "glaring defects and extreme lack of fire protection facilities." The state legislature budgeted an additional $109 million to purchase land, construct new facilities, and maintain existing facilities. Napa State Hospital was slated for complete reconditioning, which meant demolition of the Castle. Politics in the capital delayed construction, and when bids were sent out, construction companies declined, stating they did not have enough workers or materials because of the war. (Courtesy CSA.)

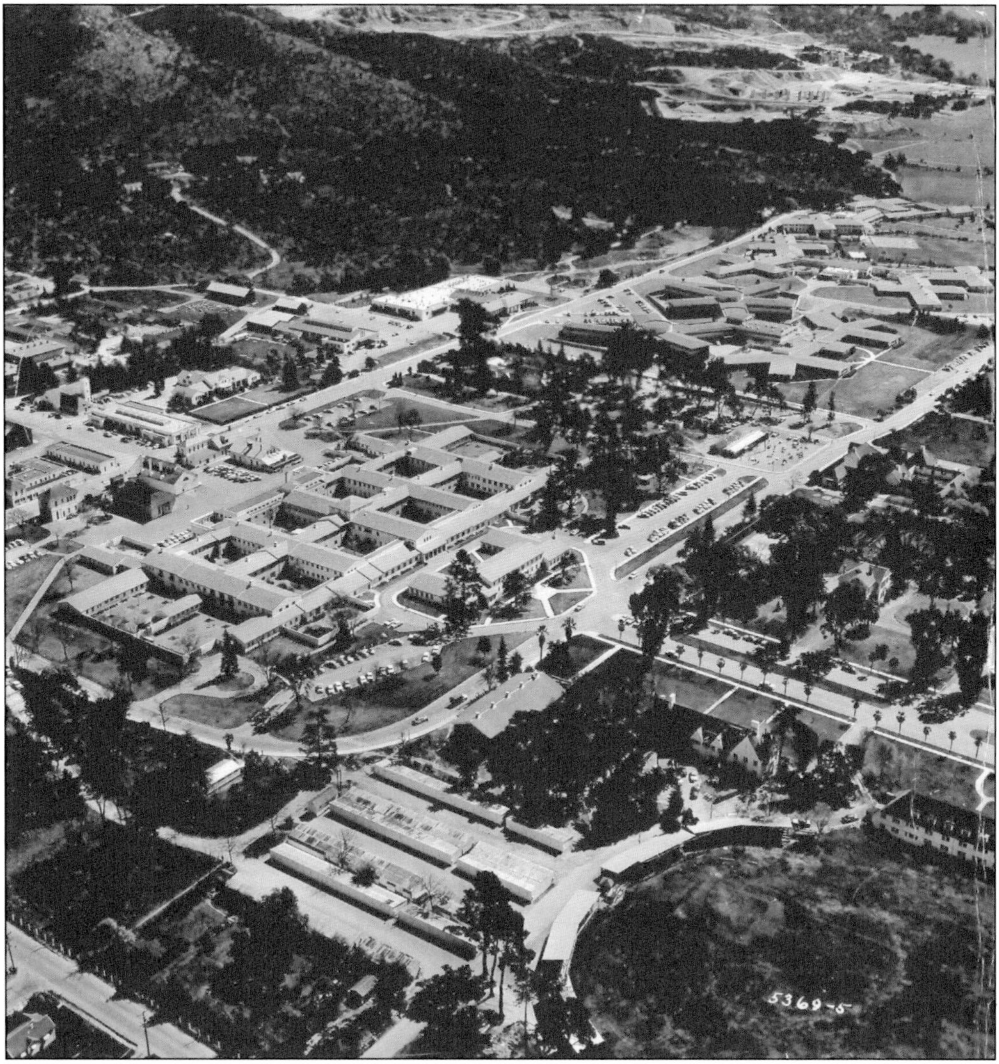

The T Units, pictured in the upper right, were a $15 million program that was launched with a ground-breaking ceremony on March 5, 1948. It was planned as 18 buildings that, when completed, would make Napa State Hospital one of the largest institutions in California. They were located south of and adjacent to the S and Q Units. The T Units were one-story buildings with courtyards and a baseball diamond. (Courtesy NCHS.)

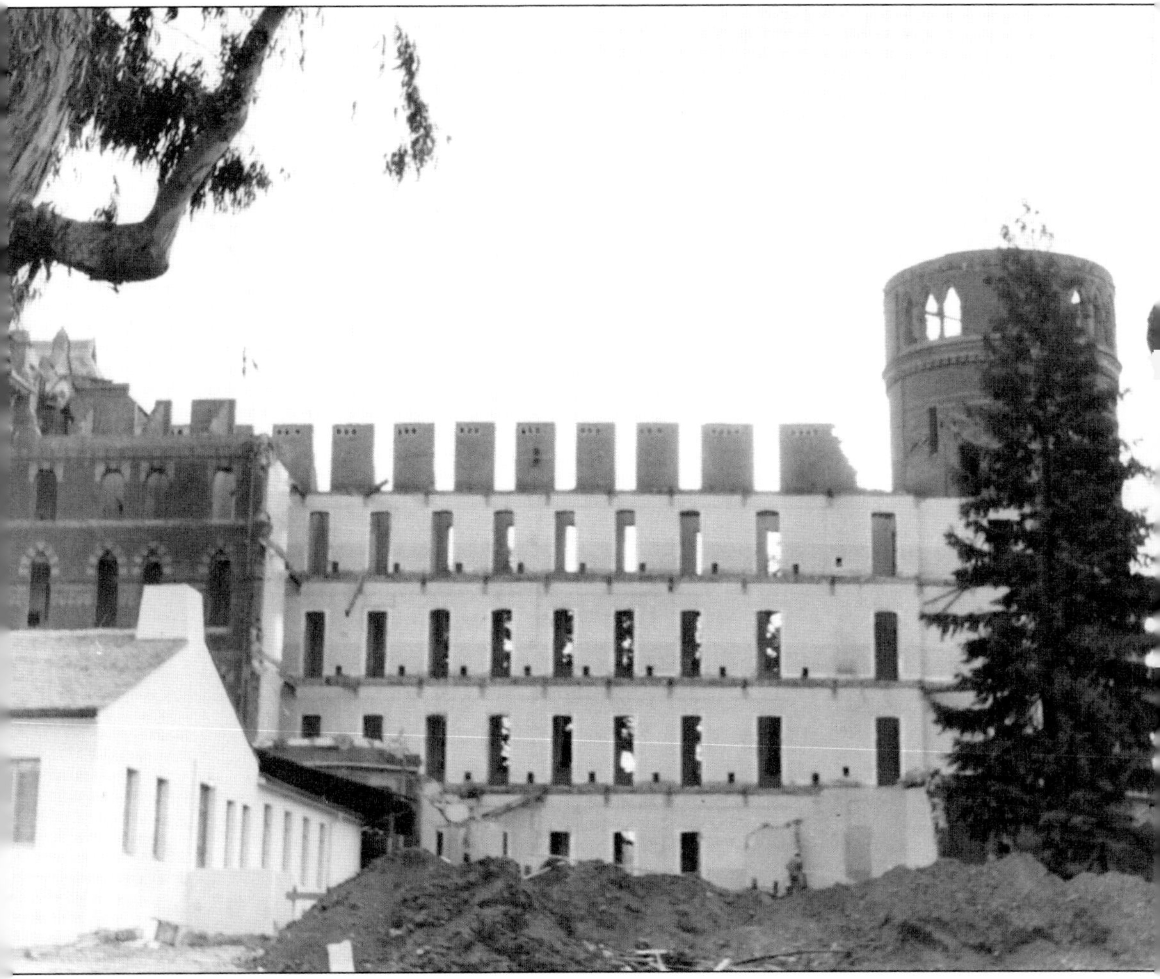

Pictured here is the demolition of the south side of the Castle. In the lower left corner is the new administration building. (Courtesy NSH.)

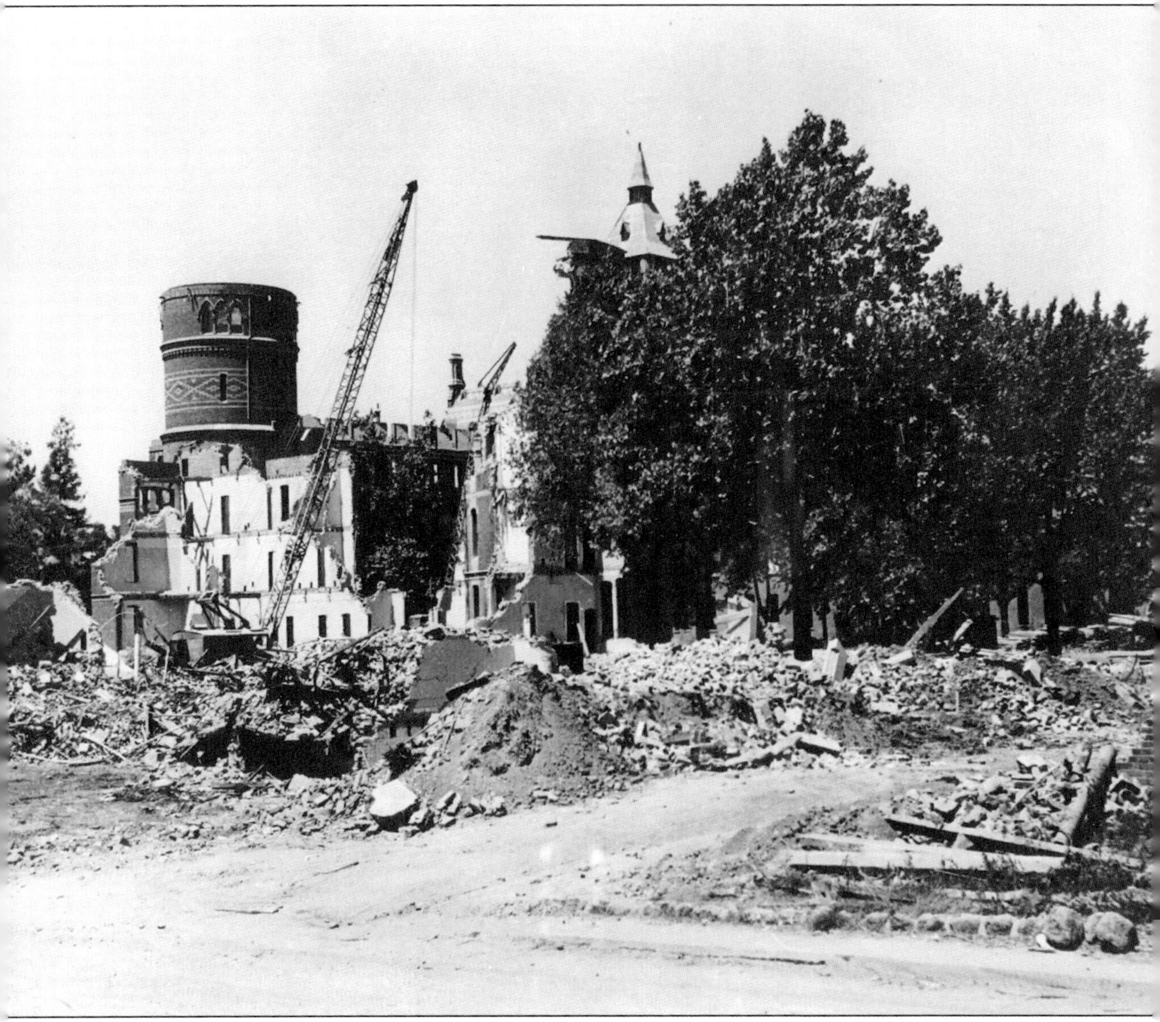

Demolition began in June 1950. Without blueprints for the underground plumbing and pipelines, rerouting of utilities became a "project of major proportions." Wrecking crews worked for 60 days until only the five-story central building was left. A large clamshell crane demolished the upper walls in three sections. When they were finished, the 10,000-gallon iron water-storage tank was visible. (Courtesy NSH.)

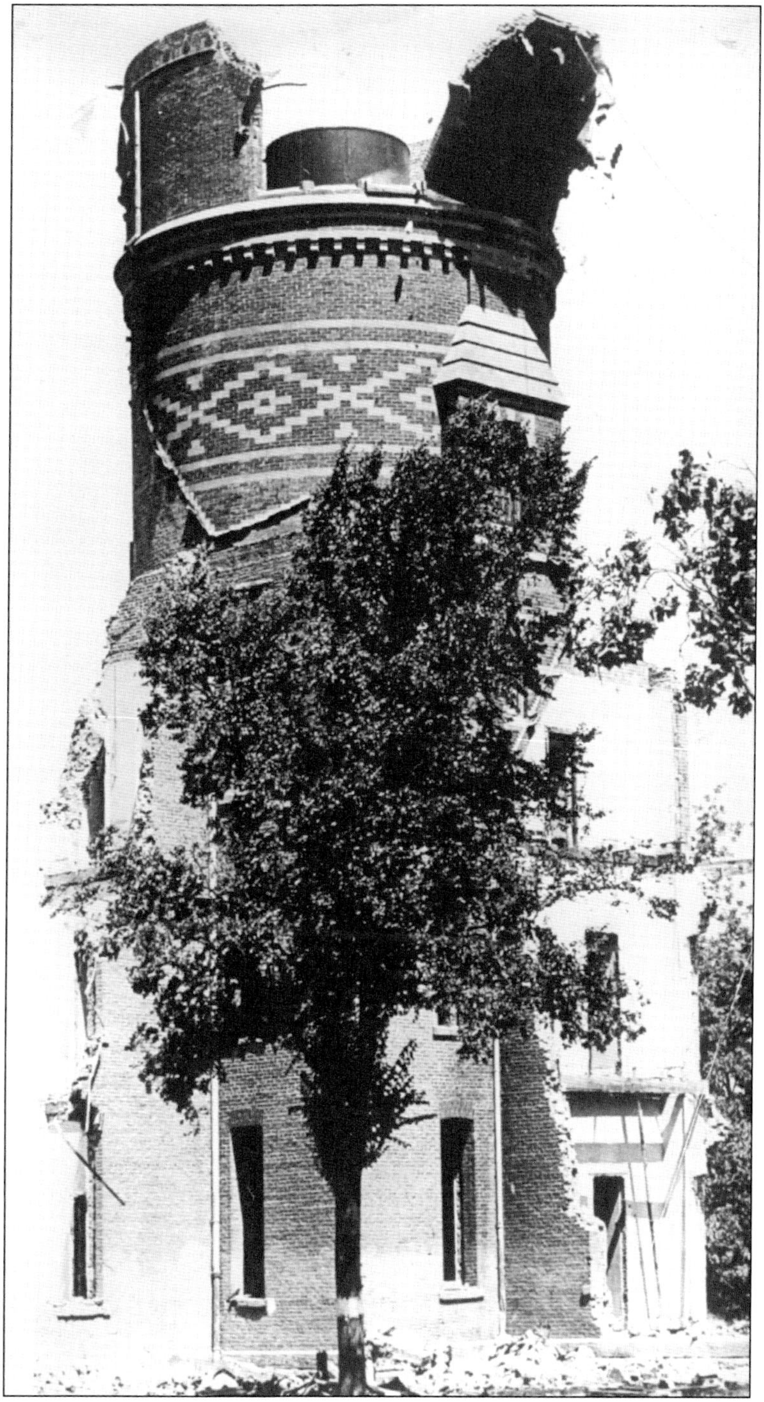

The clamshell crane was then used to lift workmen to the top of each of the four water towers, where they attached cables to the tanks and lowered them to the ground. Work was stopped in August when bees living in long-unused chimneys were disturbed. Dozens of workmen were badly stung. The fireplaces were once again used for two days to smoke out the bees, whose honey was encrusted on the inner chimney walls. (Courtesy NCHS.)

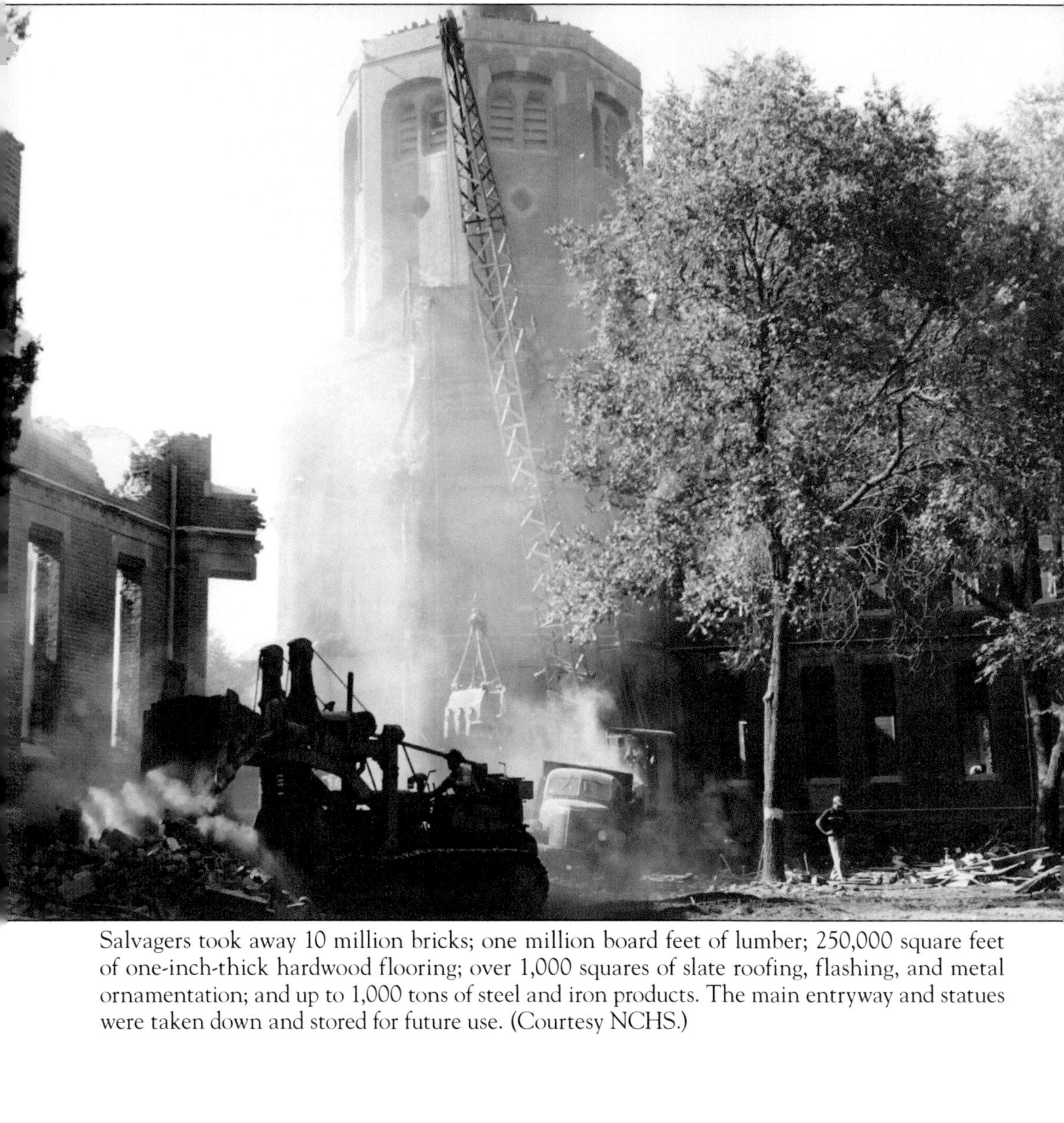

Salvagers took away 10 million bricks; one million board feet of lumber; 250,000 square feet of one-inch-thick hardwood flooring; over 1,000 squares of slate roofing, flashing, and metal ornamentation; and up to 1,000 tons of steel and iron products. The main entryway and statues were taken down and stored for future use. (Courtesy NCHS.)

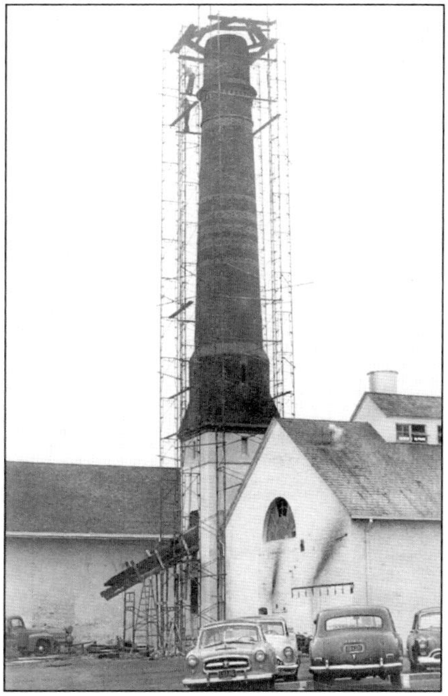

This 50-year-old chimney was used as the outlet for three boilers that provided steam heat for the Castle and outbuildings. It took about 10 days to tear down the 100,000 bricks of the 92-foot-tall chimney. (Courtesy NSH.)

Partial removal of the old administration building was done to make room for the new administration structure. The two 70-year-old magnolia trees in front survived the demolition and the construction of the new administration building. (Courtesy NSH.)

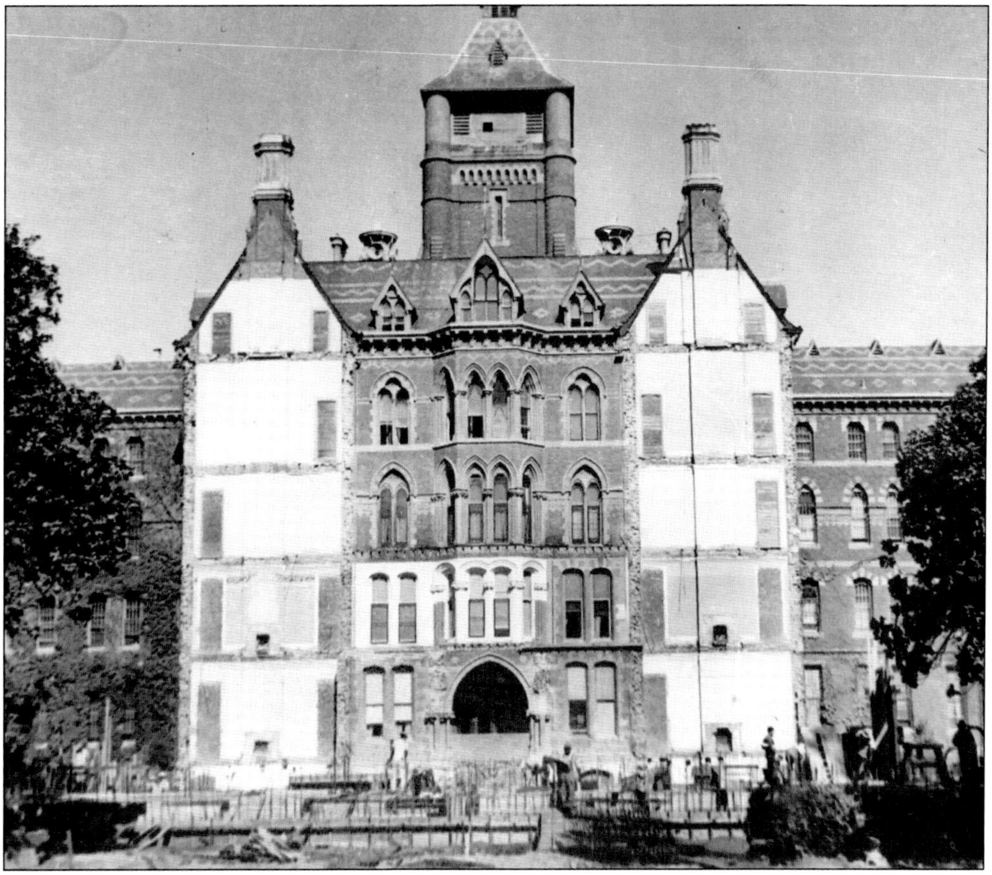

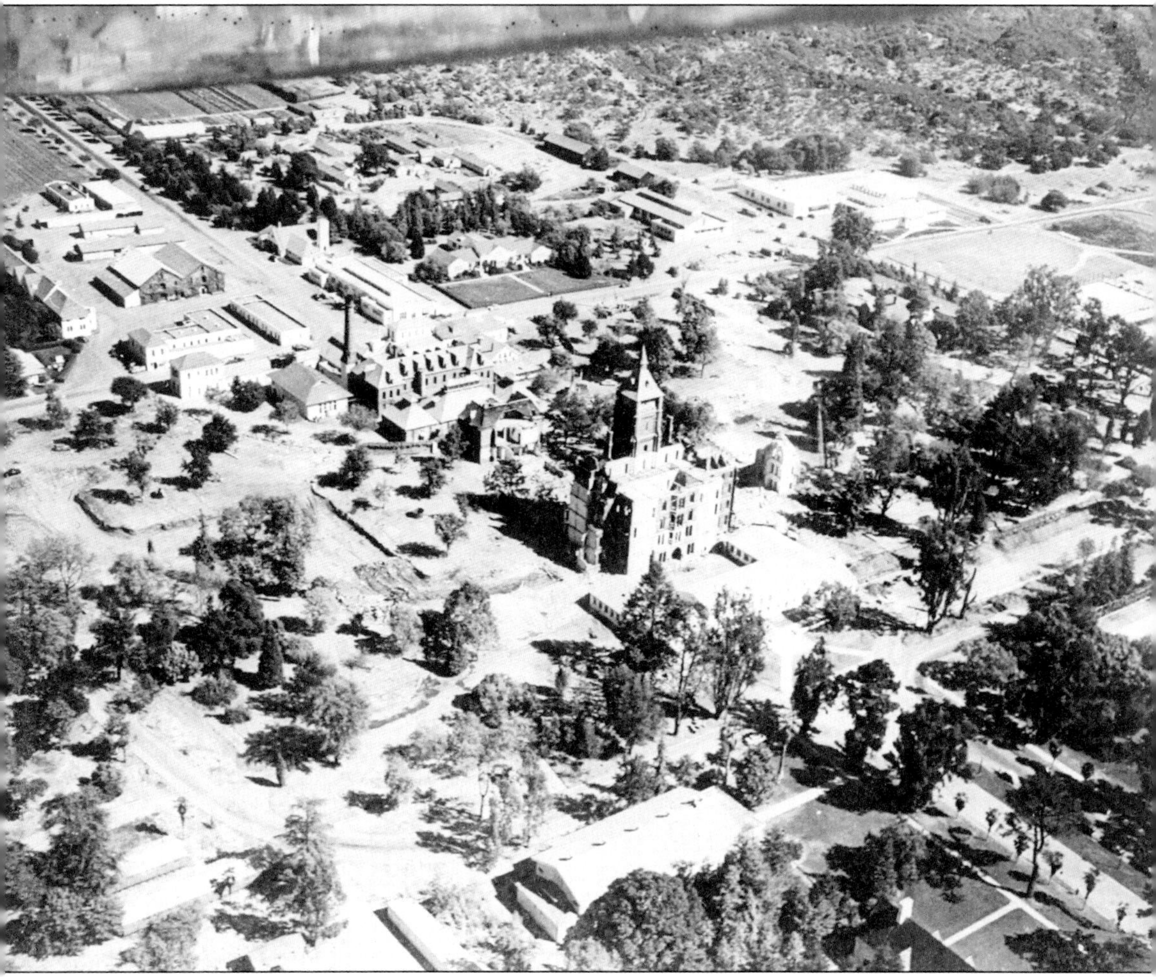

The new administration building sits directly in front of the Castle. The new treatment facility was built on the Castle site. Visible in this photograph are the remaining kitchen, chapel, and library structures. (Courtesy NSH.)

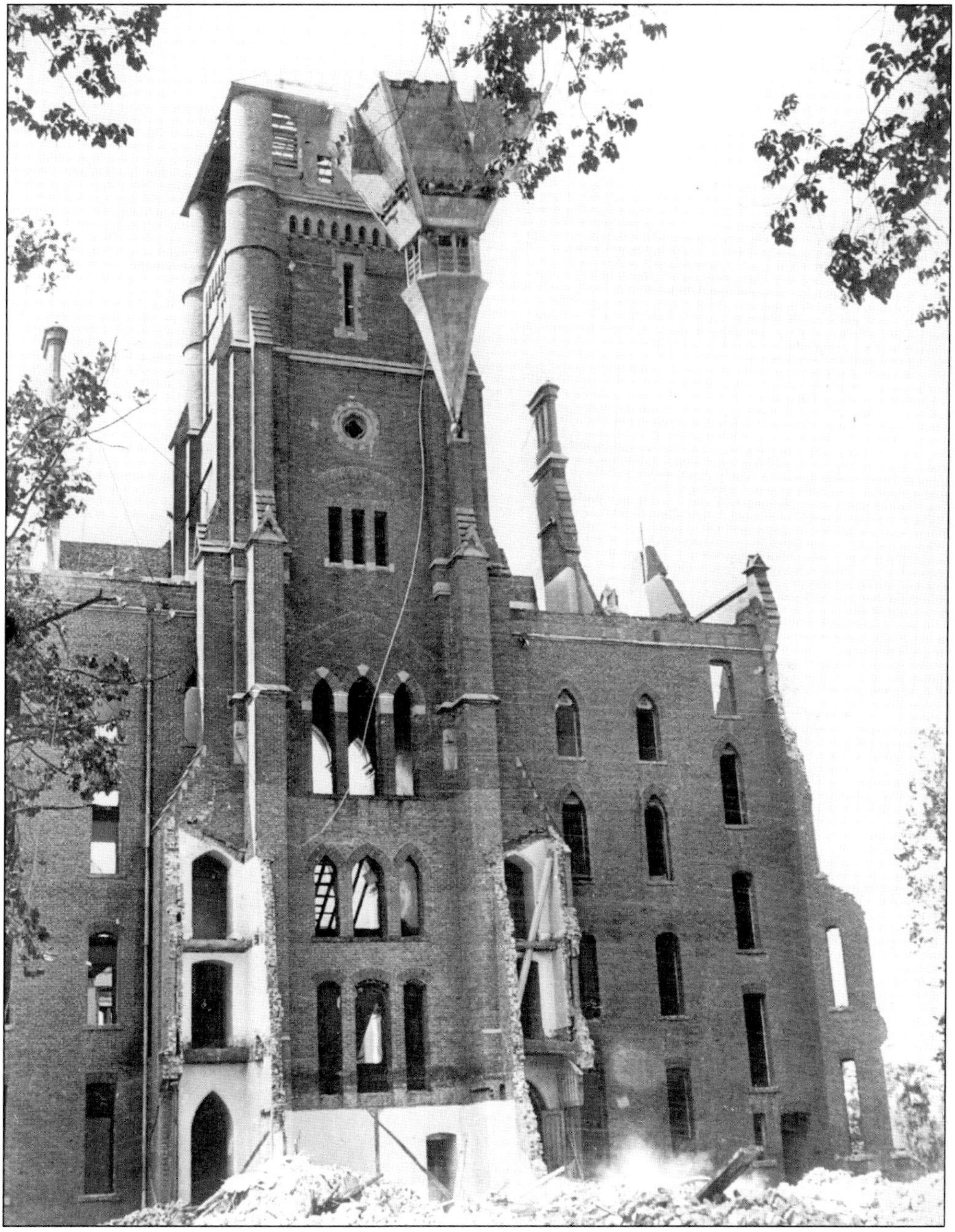

A report from a 1949 newspaper on the tower's demolition stated, "Four attempts were made to pull down the ornamental wooden tower-tip and each time the heavy cable broke. On the fifth try, it was loosened from its moorings, tilted and then fell point downward in a graceful arc before crashing to earth in a pile of splinters." (Courtesy NSH.)

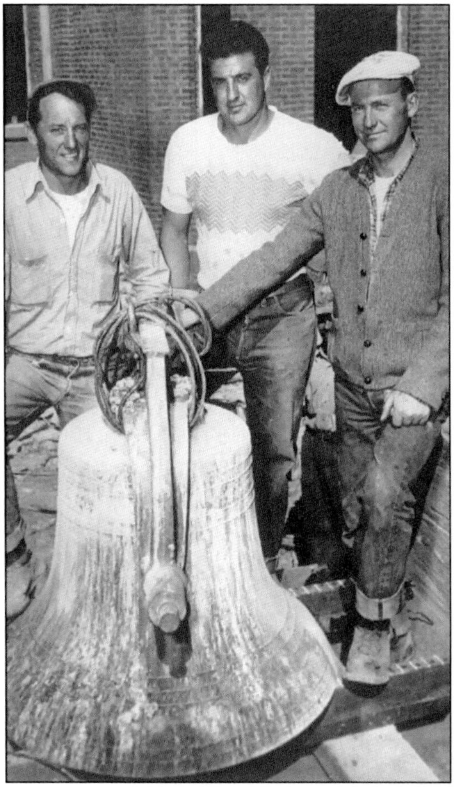

The iron bell was then lowered from the tower using a cable to bring it within reach of the clamshell crane. Cast in 1875, the bell measured three feet in diameter, two feet high, and four inches thick, with a weight of 1,800 pounds. (Courtesy NSH.)

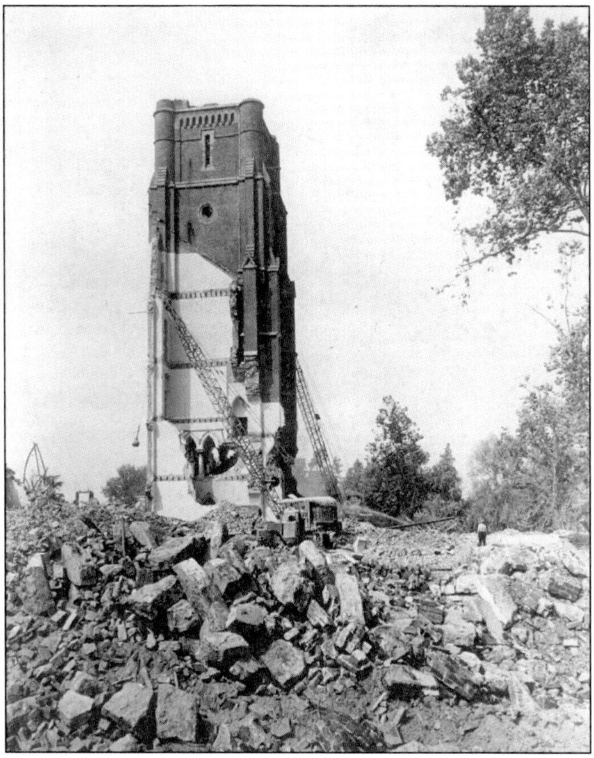

The central tower weighed 3,000 tons with solid brick walls that were eight feet thick on the second floor. Residents and employees, some with cameras, gathered in the morning and stayed all day to observe the tower's demolition. (Courtesy NSH.)

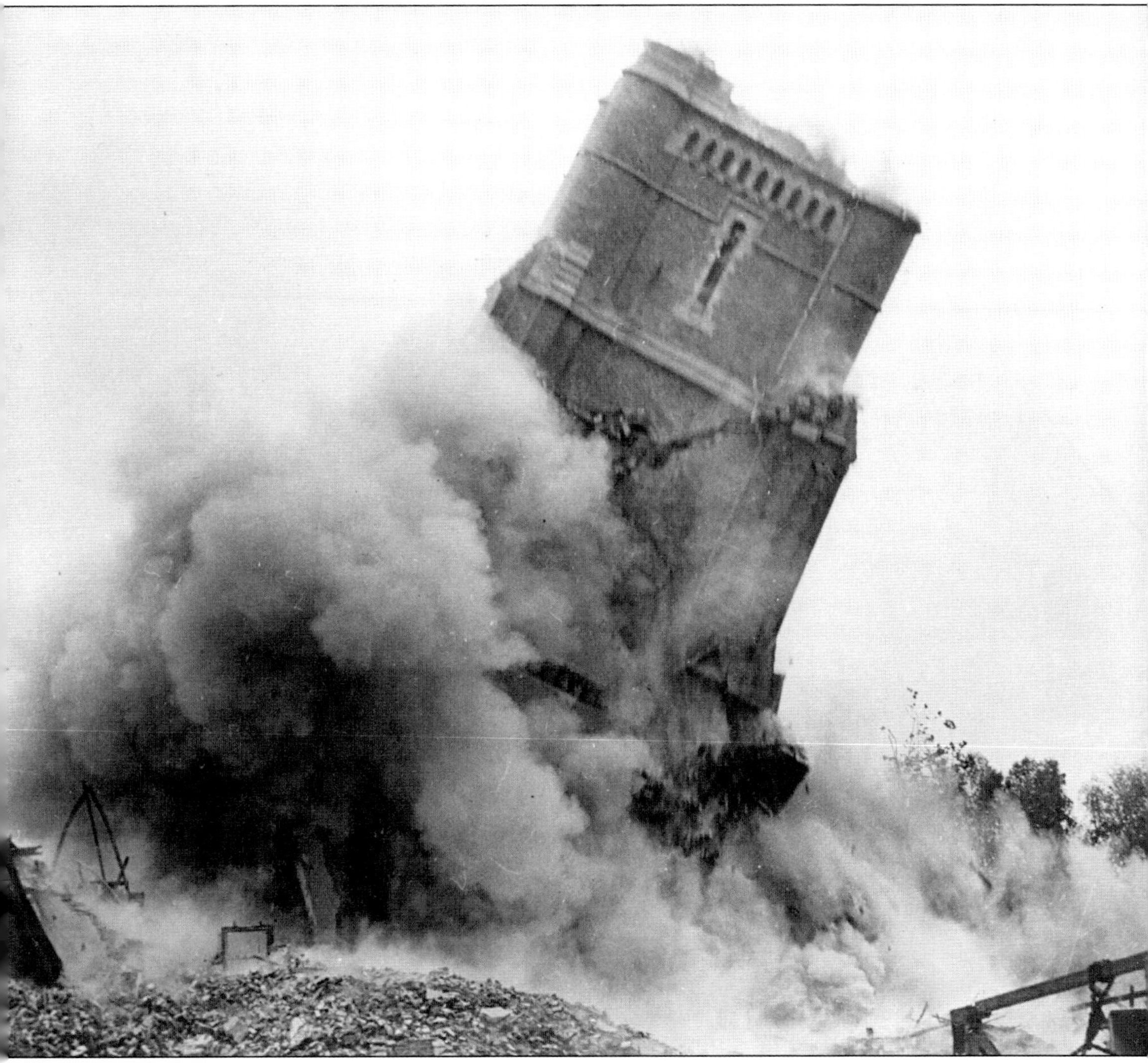

After nine hours of constant pounding with two steel wrecking balls weighing 2,300 and 3,400 pounds, the tower was brought down the next morning using a large charge of dynamite. The demolition of the central tower on September 23, 1950, has stood as the symbol for the end of the "snake pit" era for California state hospitals. (Courtesy NSH.)

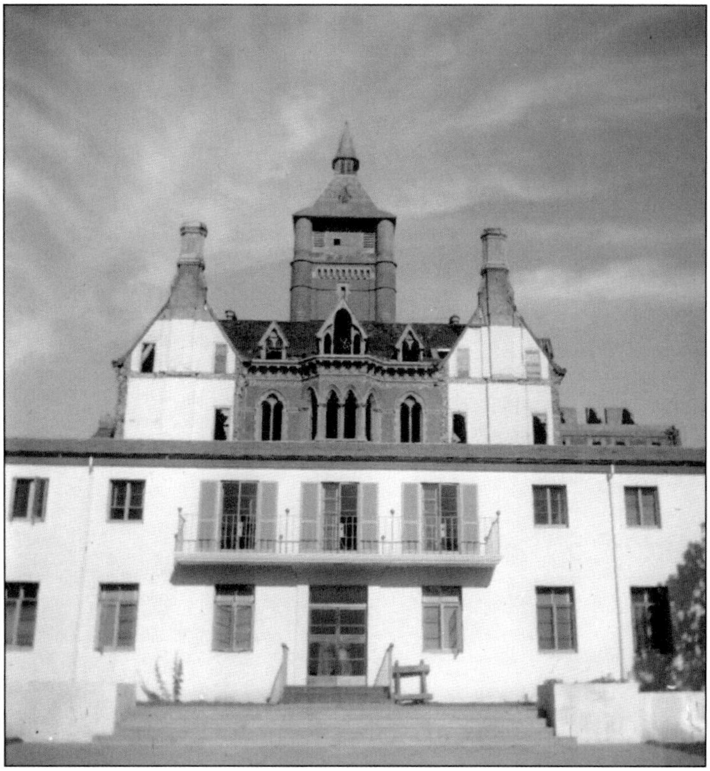

The new administration building, in front of the remains of the Castle administration wing, is pictured here in 1950. The dynamite used to demolish the central tower blew out the brand-new windows of the new administration building. (Courtesy NSH.)

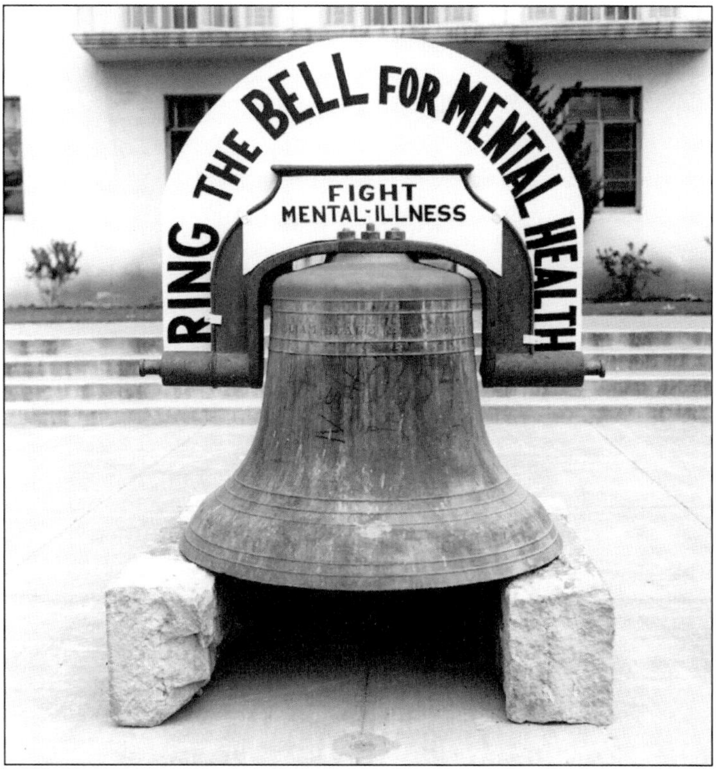

The bell was originally used to alert residents when a patient had gone missing. It was also used as a signal for the volunteer firefighters in case of fire or other emergencies. (Courtesy NSH.)

Four

A New Era 1950–1975

The new Receiving and Treatment Facility offered the promise of modern medicine combined with the latest technology available in post–World War II America. Therapy, group therapy, and social activities were combined with traditional work therapy in an effort to give patients the skills to reintegrate into their communities.

Changes in state and federal funding led to the closure of the dairy and sale of pastureland and orchards. By 1967, the dairy was no longer economically advantageous, and some of the herd was moved to Mendocino State Hospital. Psychotropic drugs and advances in the uses of antibiotics eliminated the need for long-term commitment. Community programs funded through counties aimed to provide support for discharged patients and replaced the state hospital model. Civil rights battles waged in the 1960s extended to mental illness and the disabled, which ultimately led to wide acceptance of de-institutionalization, which many believe ended the abuse and neglect that equated psychiatric hospitals with imprisonment and torture. Subsequently, these changes led to an increase in homelessness and significantly reduced the level of care.

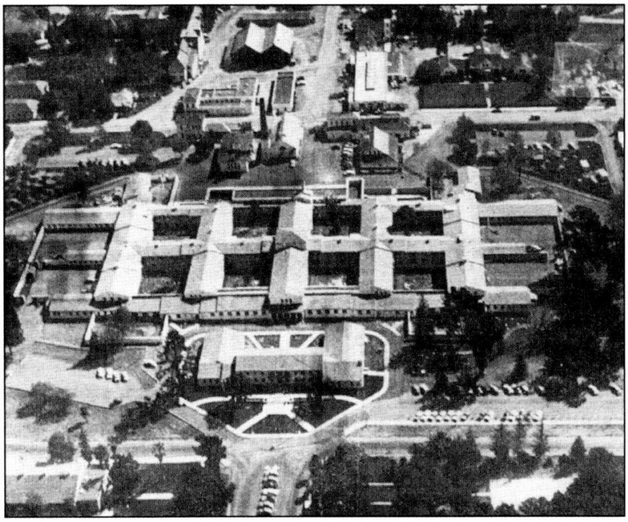

Gov. Goodwin J. Knight dedicated the new $4.5 million Napa State Hospital Receiving and Treatment (R&T) Center on December 12, 1954. Built of structurally reinforced concrete with a stucco finish, the new building was two stories high with a finished basement. There were over 300 structures on the hospital grounds at this time, including ward buildings, maintenance shops, farm buildings, garages, doctors' homes, and residence quarters for other staff. (Courtesy NCHS.)

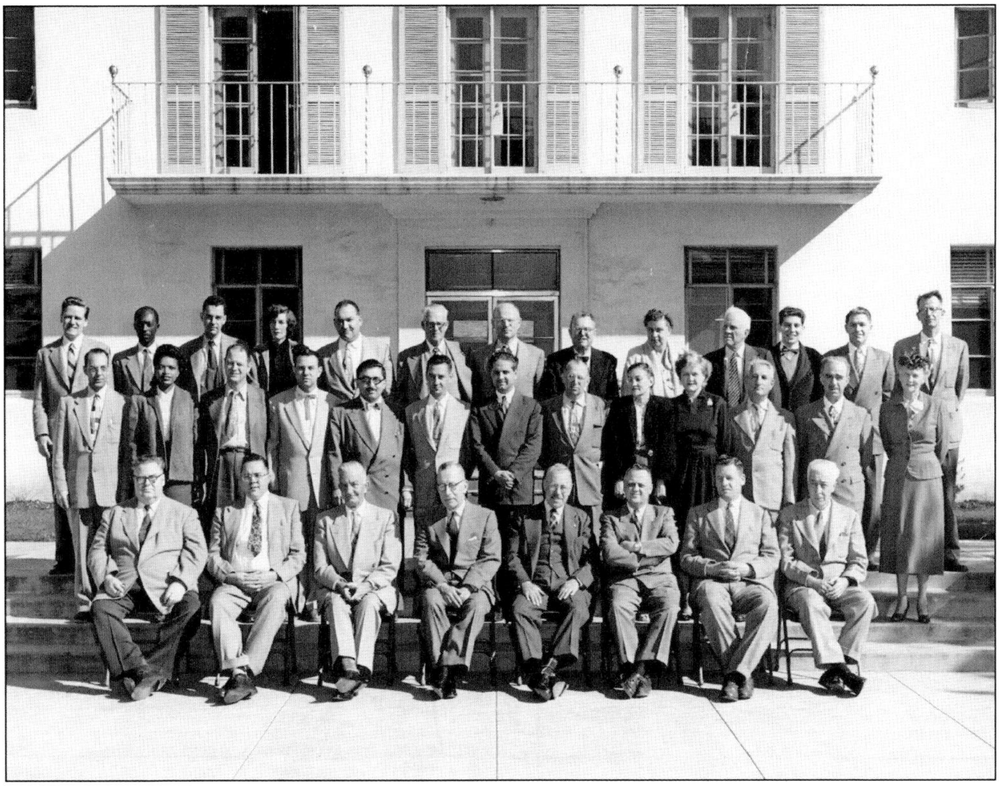

Staff physicians pose in front of the new administration building in 1955. The administrative assistant, human resources, medical records, patients' personal accounts, admission and statistical research, payroll, and other administrative functions occupied the entire south wing. In the north wing were the assistant superintendent, supervision of industries, farm management, food administration, operational and hospital property accounting, budgeting, maintenance, and fire control. The medical library, medical and ward nursing executive office, medical superintendent, and assistant medical superintendent were on the lower level. Social services and the Catholic and Protestant chaplains resided on the upper floor. (Courtesy NCHS.)

Supt. Theo K. Miller is pictured with psychiatric attendants or volunteers. Under his watch, the new facility was built and opened. (Courtesy NSH.)

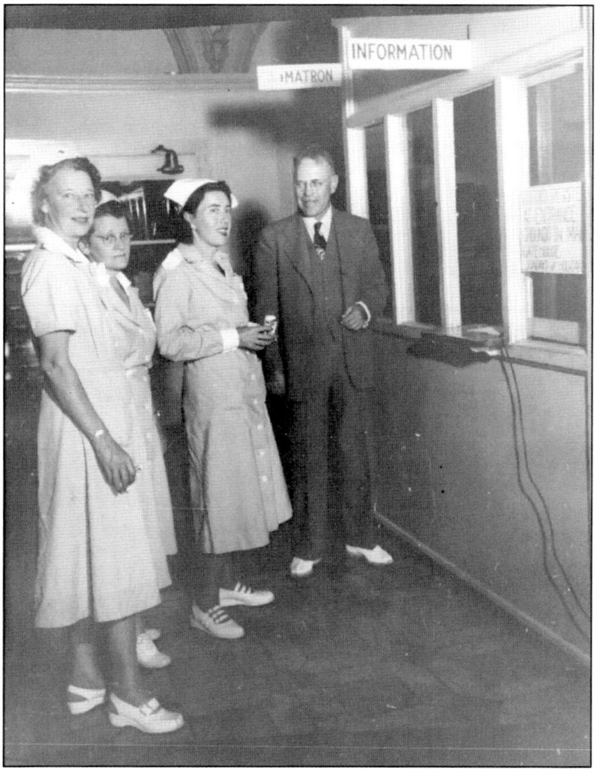

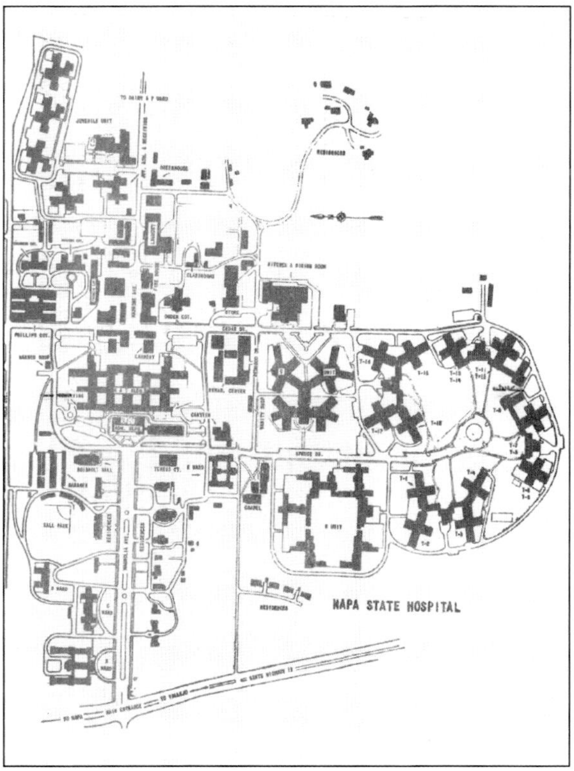

One of the few available maps of the entire property shows the layout of the facility with the completed S, Q, and T Units on the right; these were locked wards used to house patients. Treatments were undertaken in the new treatment facility seen left of center. (Courtesy NSH.)

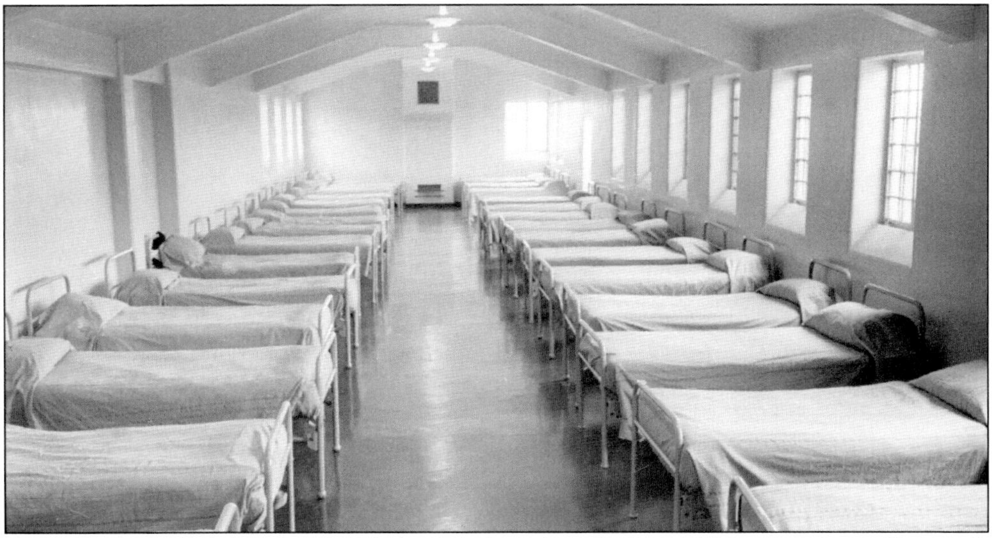

The new facility had 600 rooms, including single and two-bed rooms for patients as well as wards with 4 to 35 beds, accommodating a total of 714 patients. Each room was painted in two or more colors, from pastels to deep tones, with approximately 39 color combinations carefully chosen for their therapeutic value. This is a typical ward in the S Unit complex. (Courtesy NSH.)

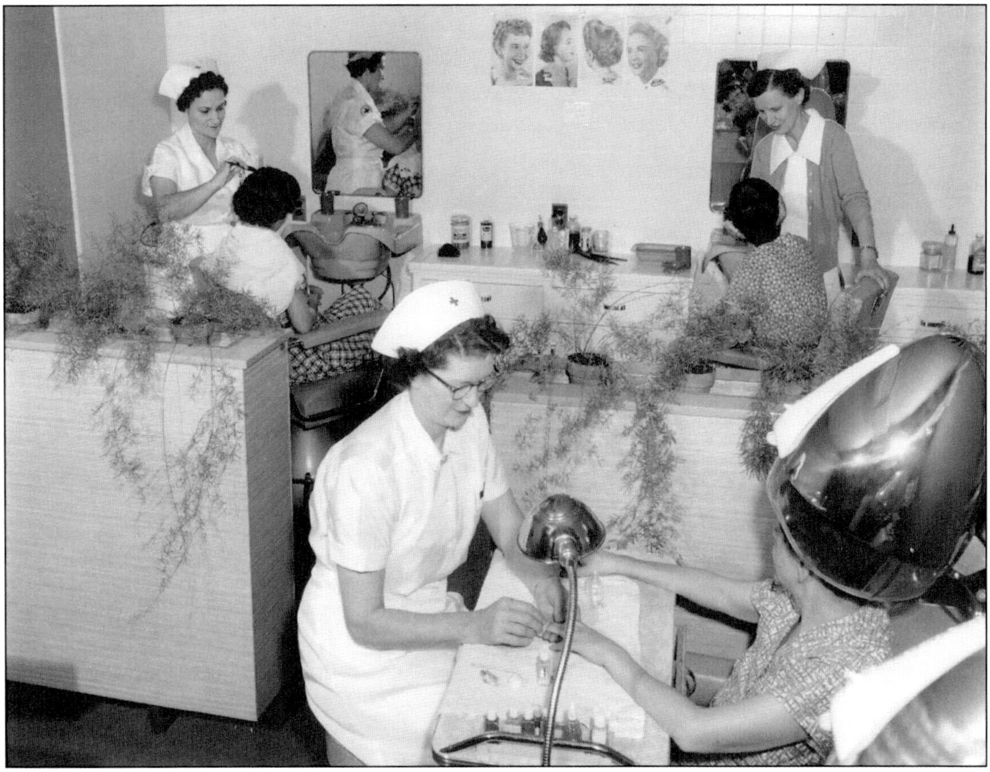

Female patients could receive regular salon services, including shampoos, finger waves, manicures, and permanent waves, as prescribed by the ward physician. The work was done by a staff of patients under the direction of a cosmetician or beauty shop manager. A psychiatric technician assisted and escorted the patients to and from the shop, which was adjacent to the Canteen. (Courtesy NSH.)

Located in the new treatment center, the dental department was equipped with a laboratory, dental X-ray facility, and three operating rooms. State hospitals were required to offer complete medical care, thus clinics for optometry, dermatology, neurosurgery, gynecology, and otolaryngology (ear, nose, and throat) were established. (Courtesy NSH.)

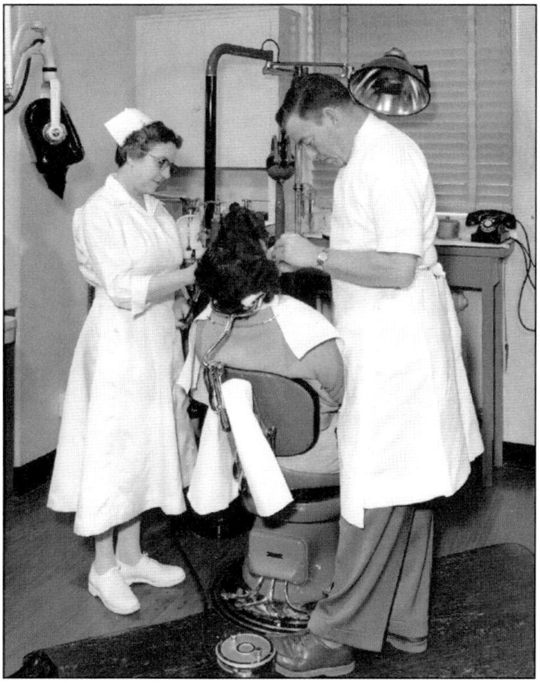

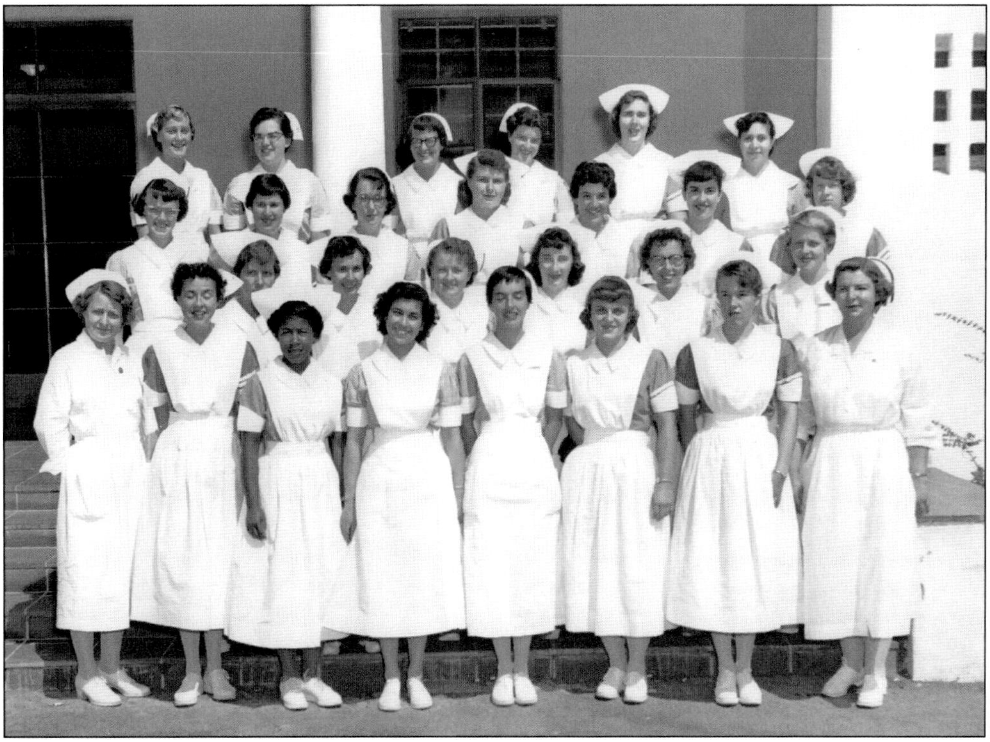

The attendants, now called psychiatric technicians, were required to have 300 hours of instruction and six months of on-the-job training before being formally approved. Formed in 1950, the California Society for Psychiatric Technicians helped to solidify a professional standard for all licensed psychiatric technicians working with mentally ill and developmentally disabled patients. (Courtesy NSH.)

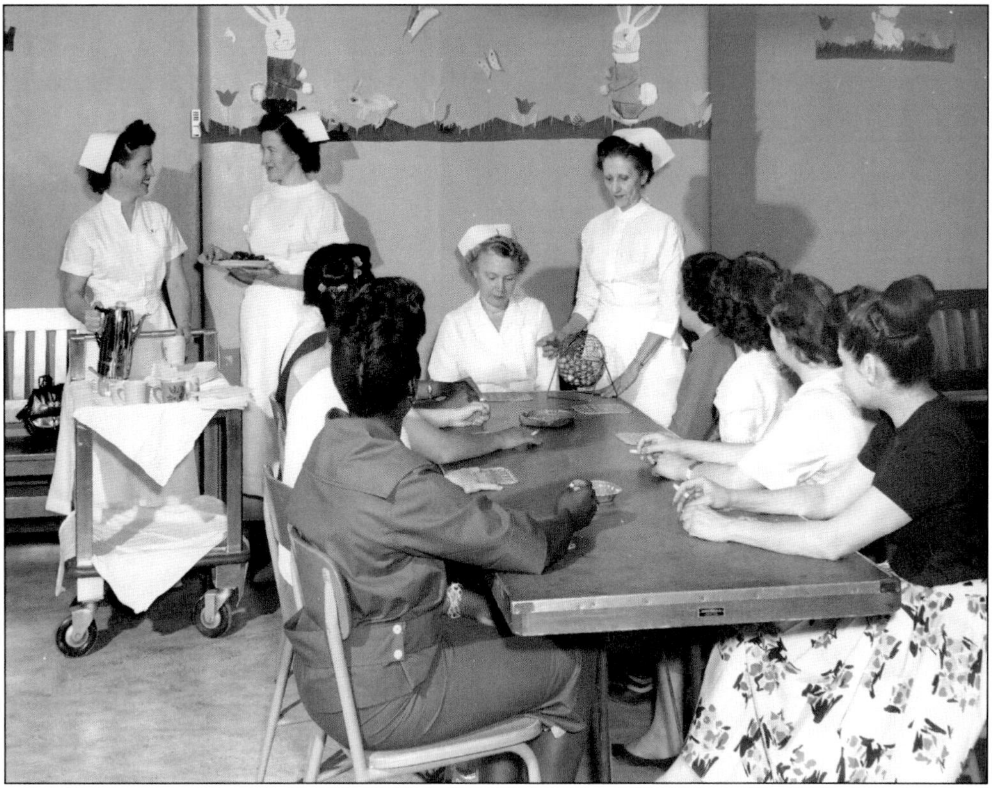

The new day-care centers provided a social and therapeutic atmosphere for patients, who could then return to their families in the evenings and on weekends. In this photograph, the patients are playing bingo. They were eligible for the same treatments as inmates: individual and group psychotherapy, relearning experiences, patient self-government, activity programs, resocialization programs, drugs, and electroshock therapy. It was located in the C Ward, near the hospital entrance on Magnolia Drive. (Courtesy NSH.)

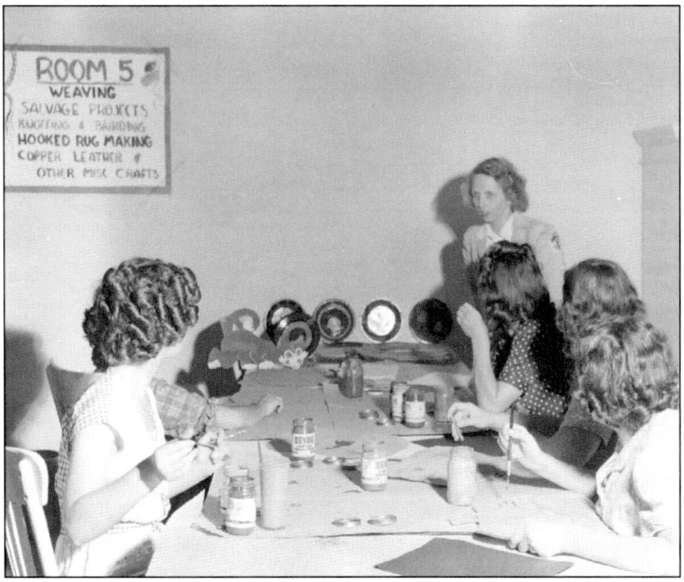
ROOM 5
WEAVING
SALVAGE PROJECTS
HOOKED RUG MAKING
COPPER LEATHER &
OTHER MISC CRAFTS

This photograph shows patients working on craft projects, such as knotting and braiding, hooked rug making, copper, leather, and other miscellaneous crafts. (Courtesy NSH.)

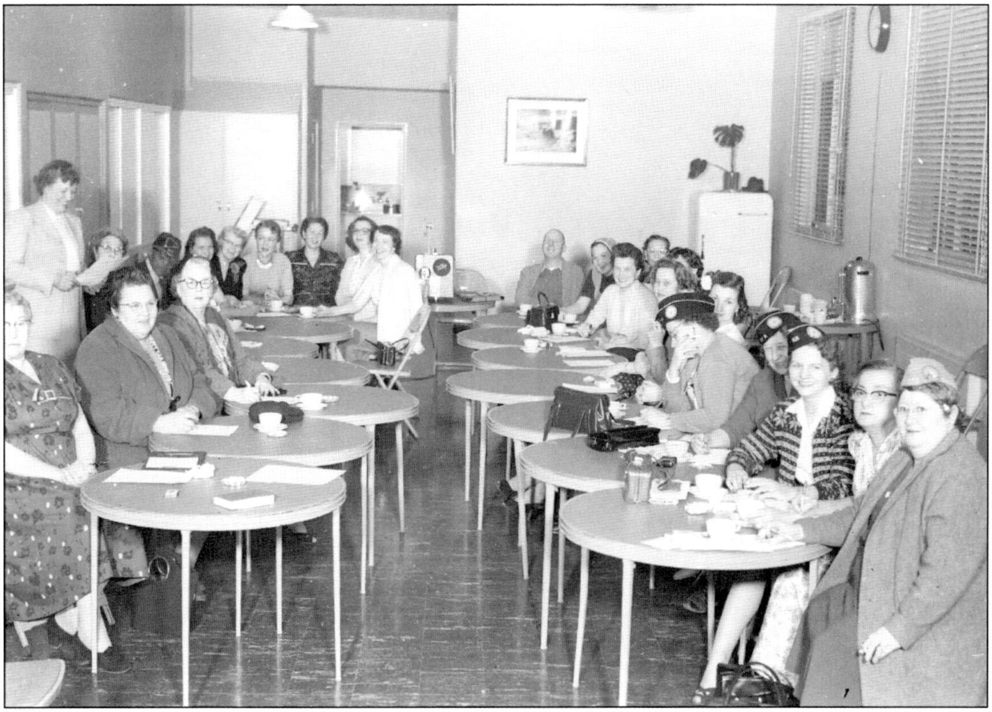

Staff and volunteers relax in the cafeteria of the new treatment center about 1950. Volunteer aid was crucial in providing personal attention to the patients. (Courtesy NSH.)

In 1954, the *Napa Register* reported that 60 volunteers from the North Bay Area chapters of the Grey Ladies of the Red Cross of America, as well as other civic groups, donated 5,300 hours of volunteer aid each month to recreational and occupational therapy projects. (Courtesy NSH.)

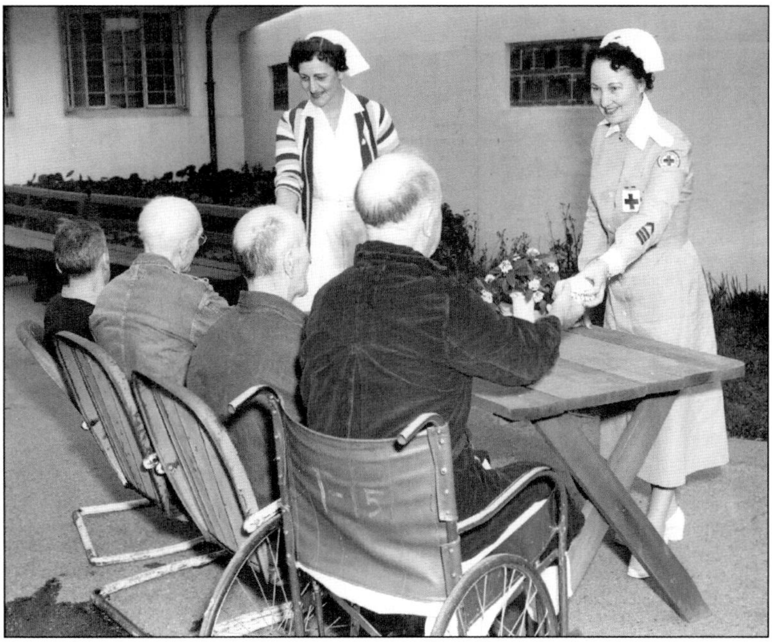

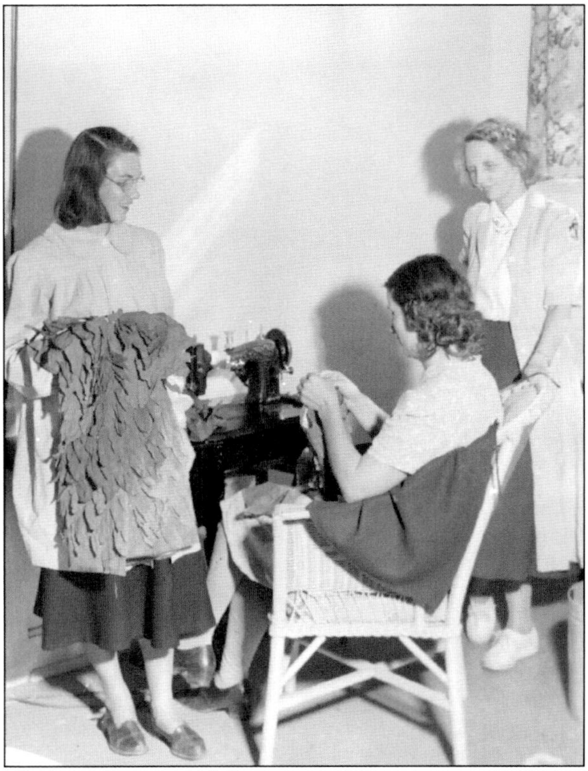

In 1954, there were 600 patients assigned to industrial and other work therapy projects around the hospital according to their abilities. Patients were offered courses in industrial work, styling of hair and clothes, cooking, ceramics, skin treatment, tennis, copper tooling, dress modeling, and practical nursing. (Courtesy NSH.)

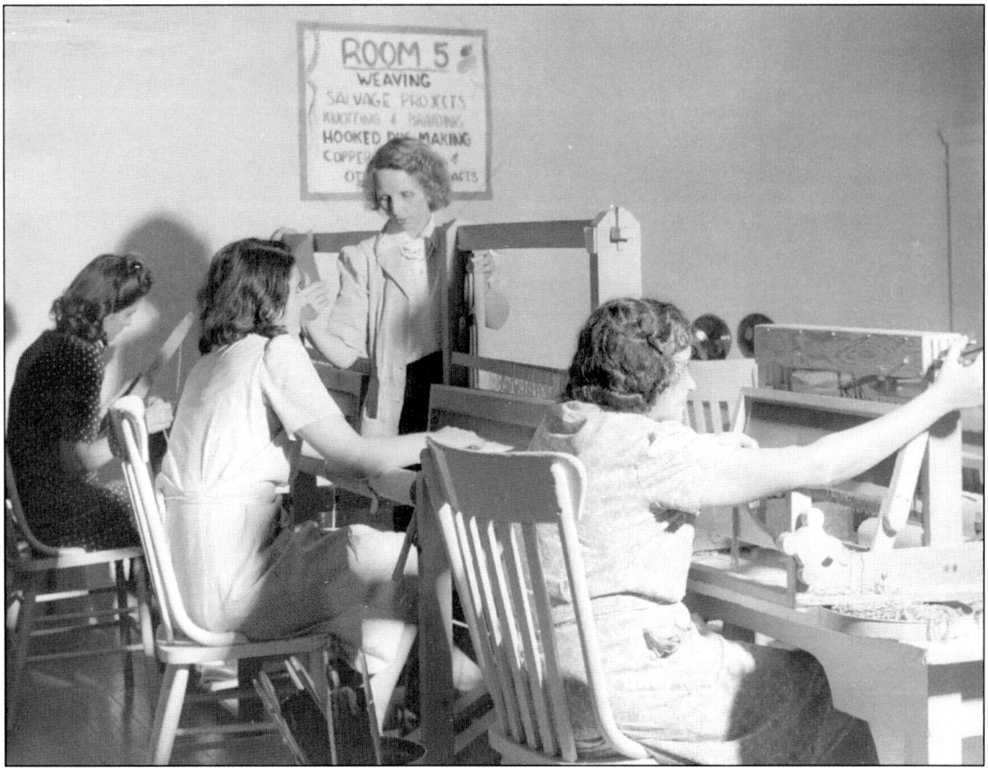

Although occupational therapy and farmwork continued as forms of treatment, individual and group therapy were emphasized, as well as contact with a social worker who would assist with a patient's transition after being discharged from the hospital. (Courtesy NSH.)

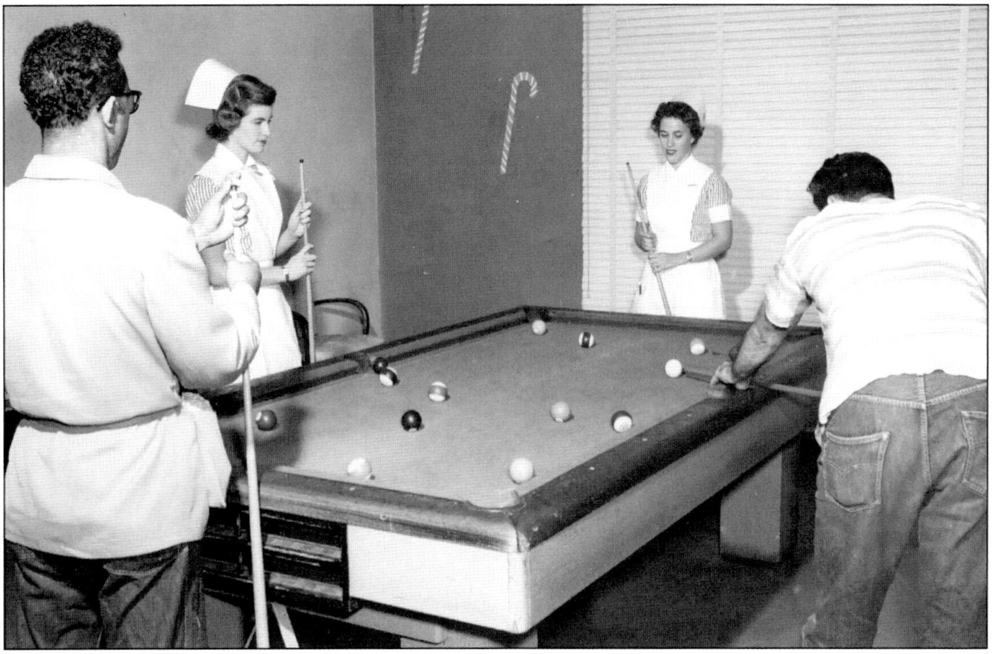

New programs included classroom work in occupational therapy, organized hikes on the grounds, visits to the Canteen, weekly movies, folk dancing classes, church services, athletic activities, community singing, ping-pong, and card games; ward parties were encouraged by the ward personnel as well. The intention was to create a cheerful and homelike atmosphere. (Courtesy NSH.)

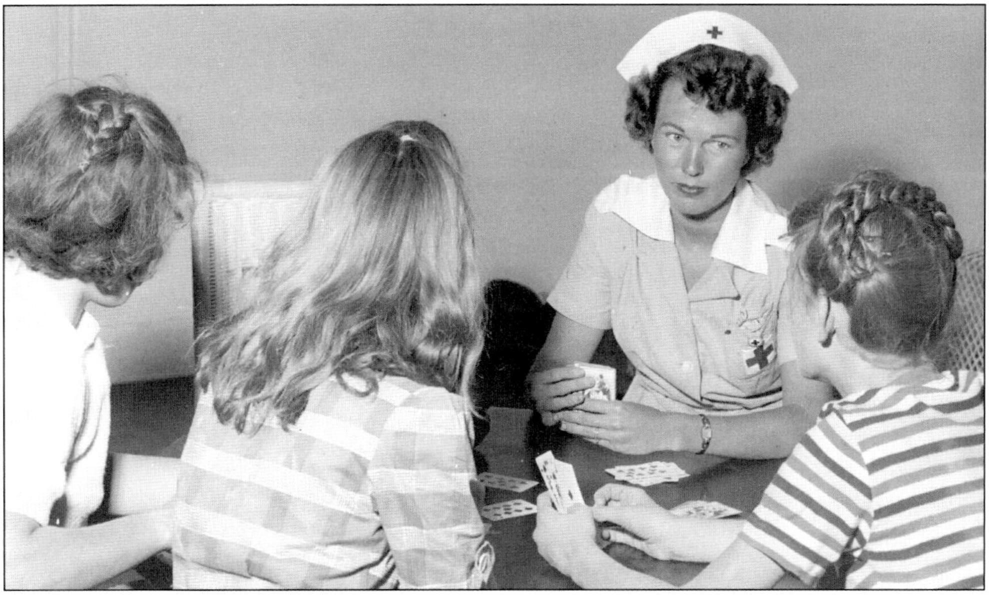

Supt. Theo K. Miller established the children's unit to meet the needs of kids referred by the Juvenile Courts or Youth Authority who had displayed atypical or violent behavior at an early age. The children's program had the highest ratio of staff to patients: one staff for every nine children. There were two part-time doctors, three teachers, a full-time psychologist, two part-time psychologists, and two full-time doctors in training. It was one of six children's programs in the United States when it opened. (Courtesy NSH.)

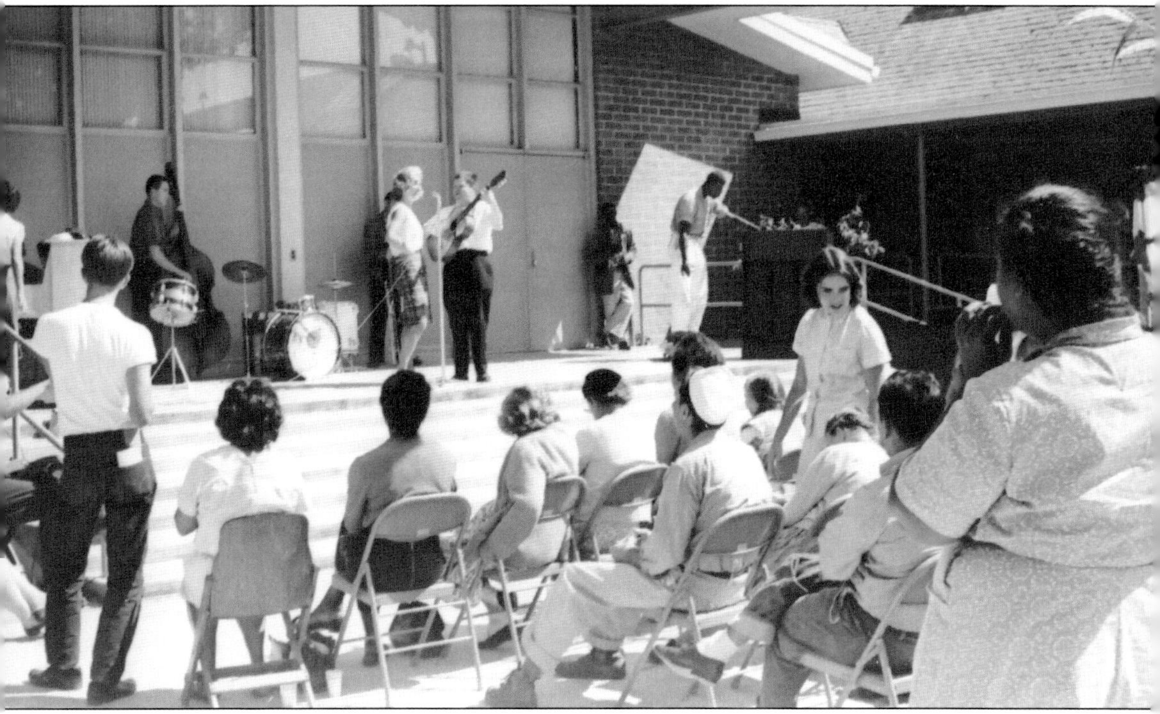

Sue Mouchka and Leland Brewster, who were rehabilitation therapists, perform a duet. (Courtesy NSH.)

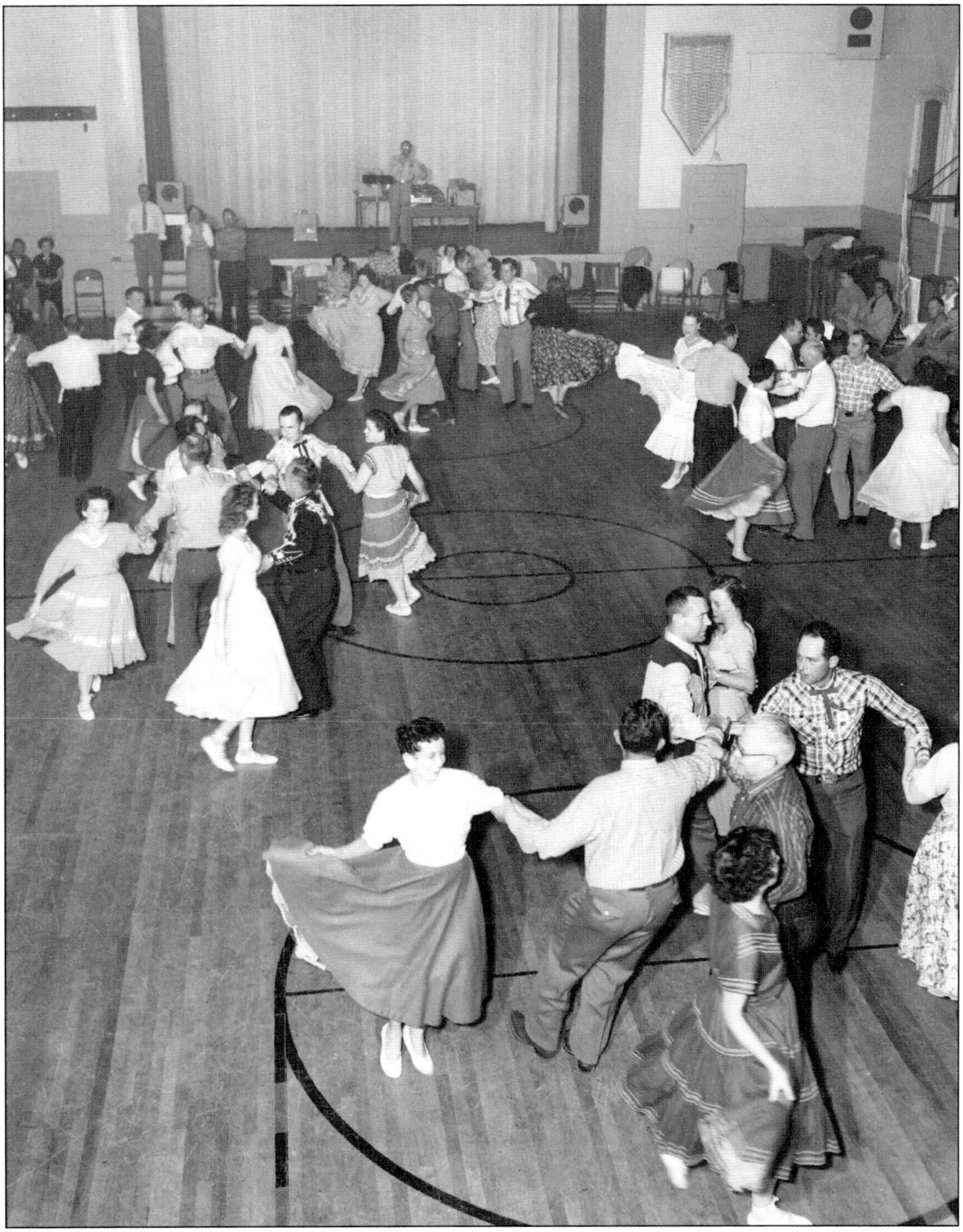

The recreational program included a square dance in Hoisholt Hall on Monday nights, a picnic on Wednesday afternoons, organized hikes around the grounds, a dance with music by a patients' orchestra on Saturday afternoons, and a community sing-along on Sunday nights, in addition to the weekly movie. (Courtesy NSH.)

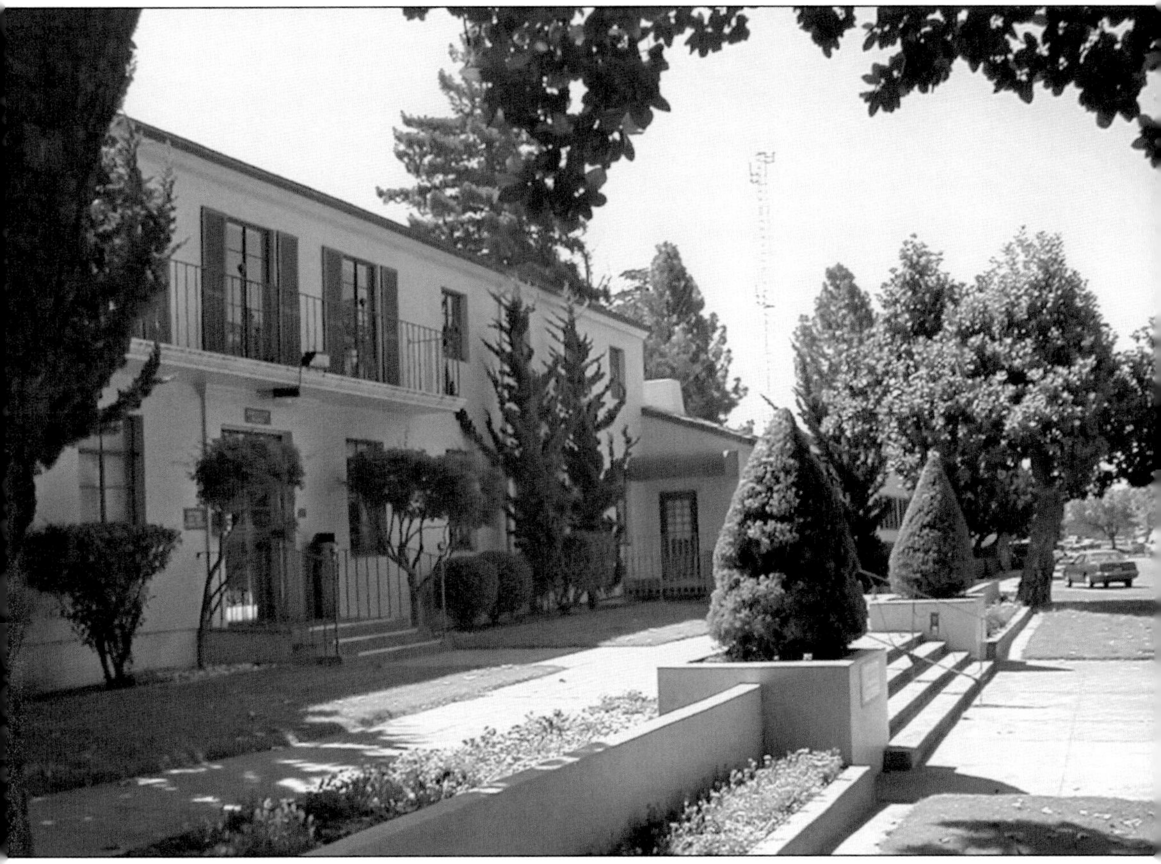

According to a 1952 *San Francisco Chronicle* interview of Dr. W.A. Oliver, director of clinical services, social activities were designed to keep patients busy with activities that help "return them to the real world and with each other. Painting, music, games and hobbies give them a chance to relieve in useful ways the pent up feelings that are basic to their illness. . . . Nearly every patient participates to some extent. An intensive combination of all of them, referred to as 'total push' is reserved for patients who have the best chances of recovery and who have been ill for the shortest time. Because of limited funds and personnel, only 160 patients out of 4,400 at the hospital are getting 'total push.' " (Courtesy NSH.)

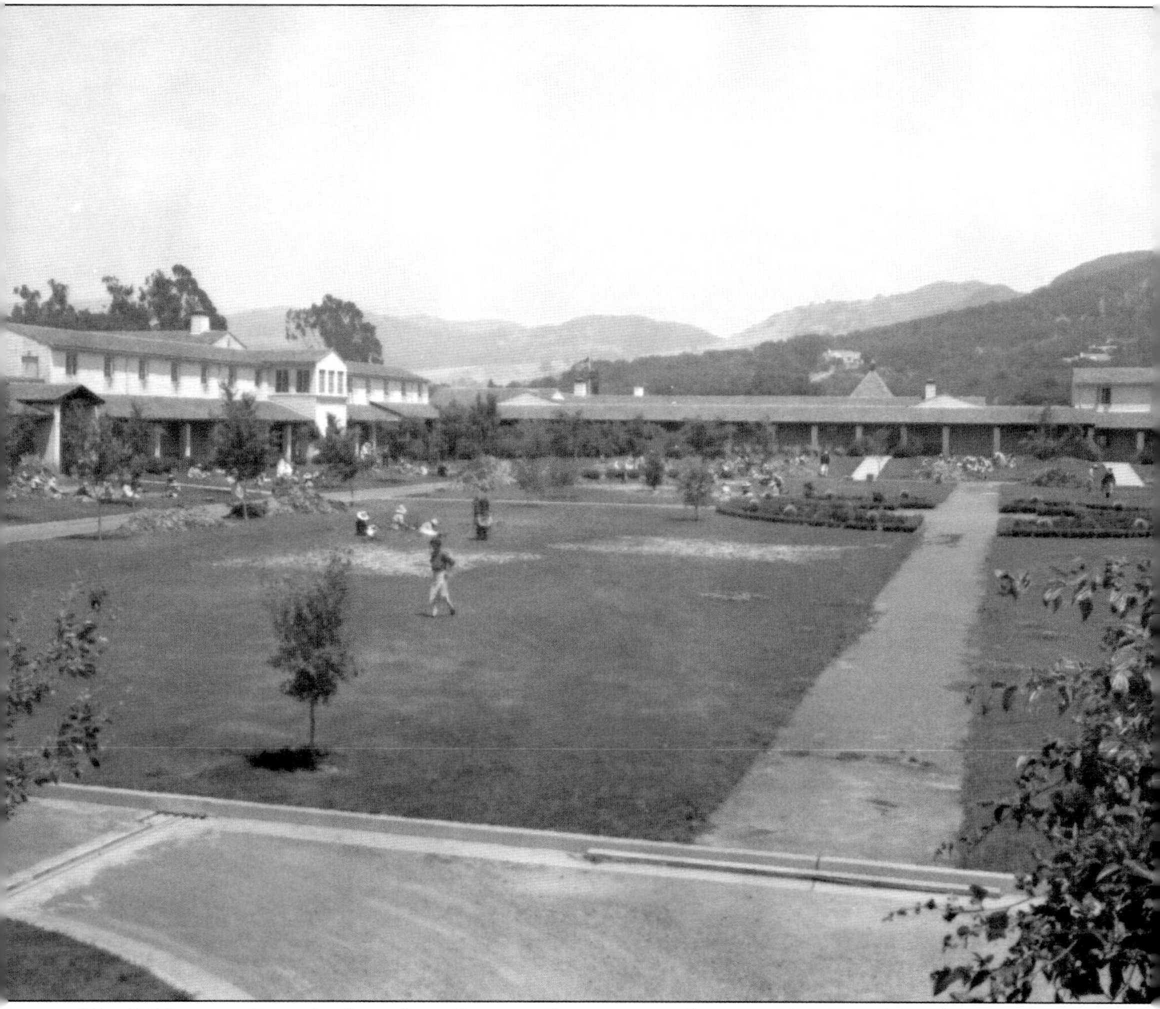

The S Unit quad was built and used primarily as patient housing. As mental health services began to shift to county services and populations declined, developmentally disabled clients were housed there. (Courtesy NSH.)

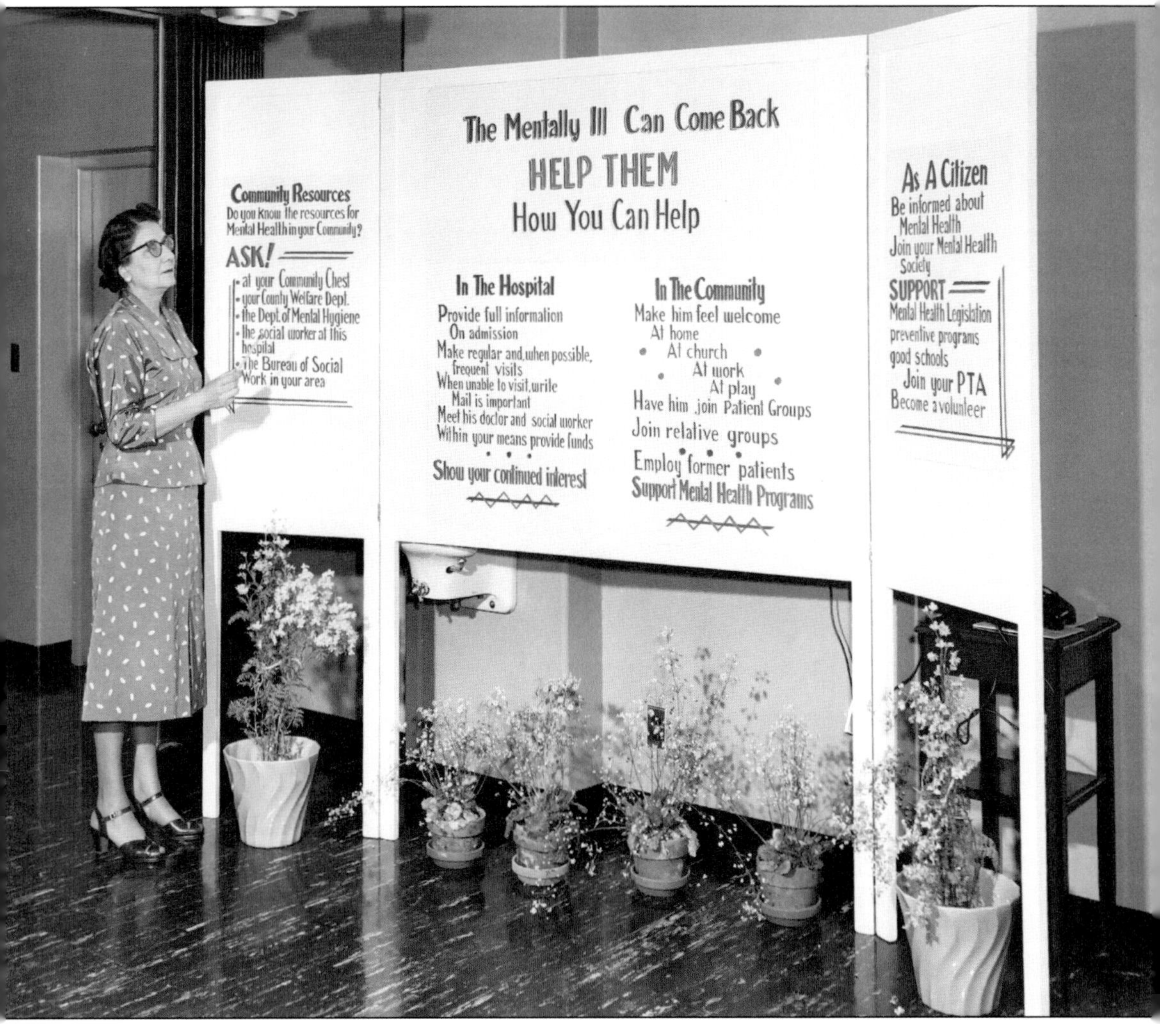
The Mentally Ill Can Come Back
HELP THEM
How You Can Help
Community Resources
Do you know the resources for Mental Health in your Community?
ASK!
at your Community Chest
your County Welfare Dept.
the Dept. of Mental Hygiene
the social worker at this hospital
The Bureau of Social Work in your area
In The Hospital
Provide full information On admission
Make regular and, when possible, frequent visits
When unable to visit, write
Mail is important
Meet his doctor and social worker
Within your means provide funds
Show your continued interest
In The Community
Make him feel welcome
At home
At church
At work
At play
Have him join Patient Groups
Join relative groups
Employ former patients
Support Mental Health Programs
As A Citizen
Be informed about Mental Health
Join your Mental Health Society
SUPPORT
Mental Health Legislation
preventive programs
good schools
Join your PTA
Become a volunteer

On April 28, 1957, the Napa State Hospital opened its doors for a weeklong open house in honor of Mental Health Week. A poster, titled "The Mentally Ill Can Come Back," made by a patient in the work therapy department was featured in the conference room of the R&T building. Approximately 200 visitors toured the hospital wards. Other events included panel discussions, films, and displays with educational material on local social services and community mental health facilities. (Courtesy NSH.)

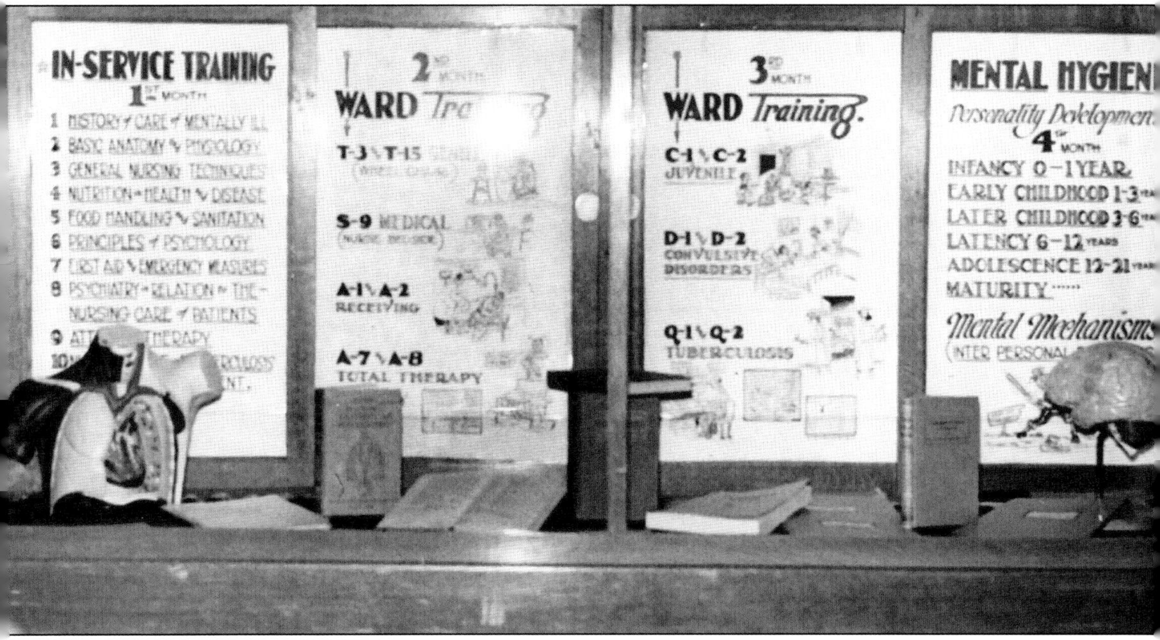

In-service educational staff included one staff nurse assigned full-time for classroom instruction and a supervising psychiatric technician. Instructors from the Napa College adult education department gave courses specially designed for state hospital medical staff in such subjects as psychiatry and neurology. Professional internships provided a 12-week field-training period for Napa College students enrolled in the vocational nurse course. (Courtesy NSH.)

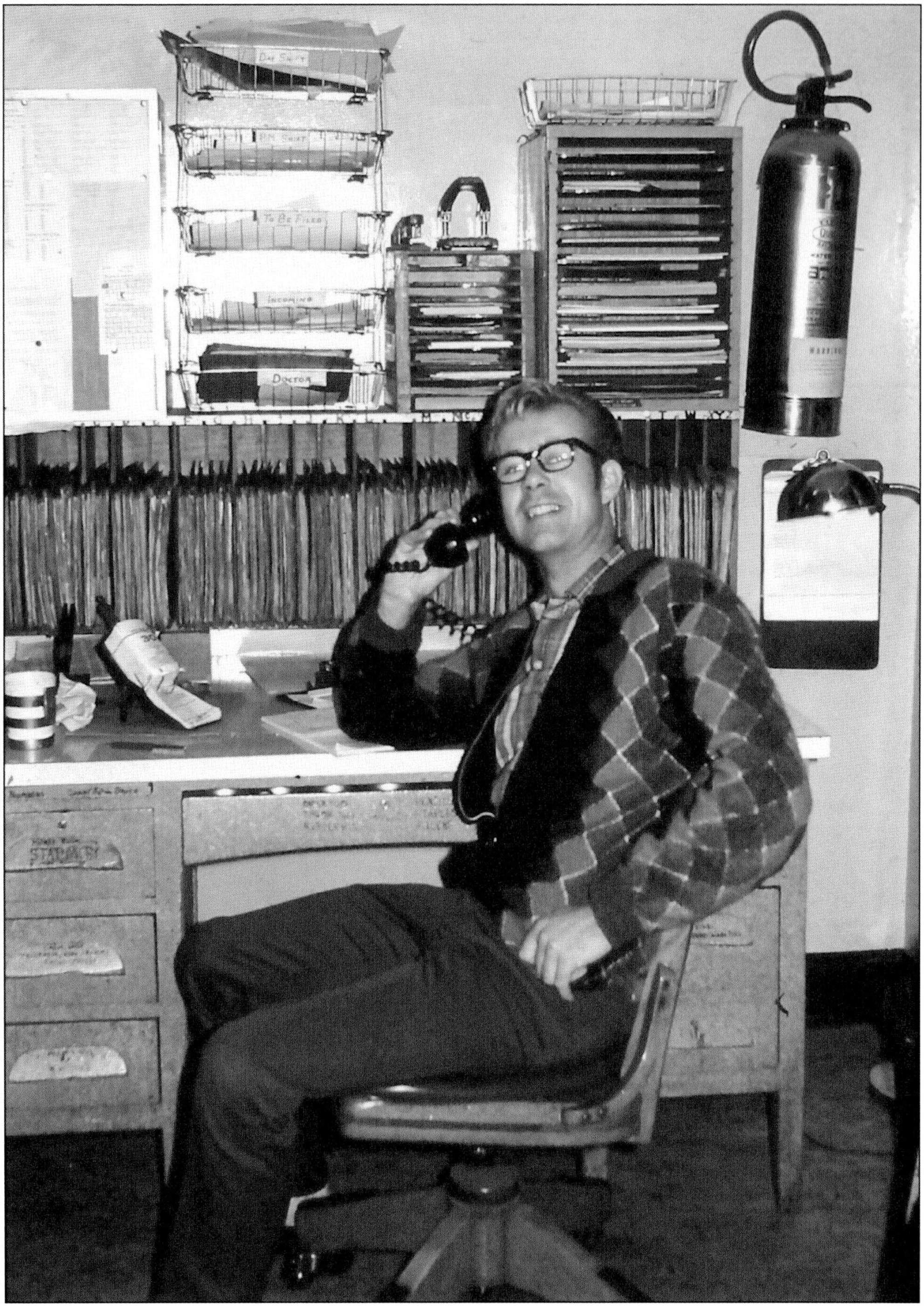

Peter Zwetsloot poses at his desk at Francis Cottage. He began working for Napa State Hospital after a year at Veteran's Hospital in Napa. He trained as a psychiatric technician and became a supervisor, managing three shifts. After a heart attack, for which doctors gave him three years to live, the Napa State Hospital transferred him into the warehouse, from where he retired after 22 years of service. (Courtesy Peter Zwetsloot.)

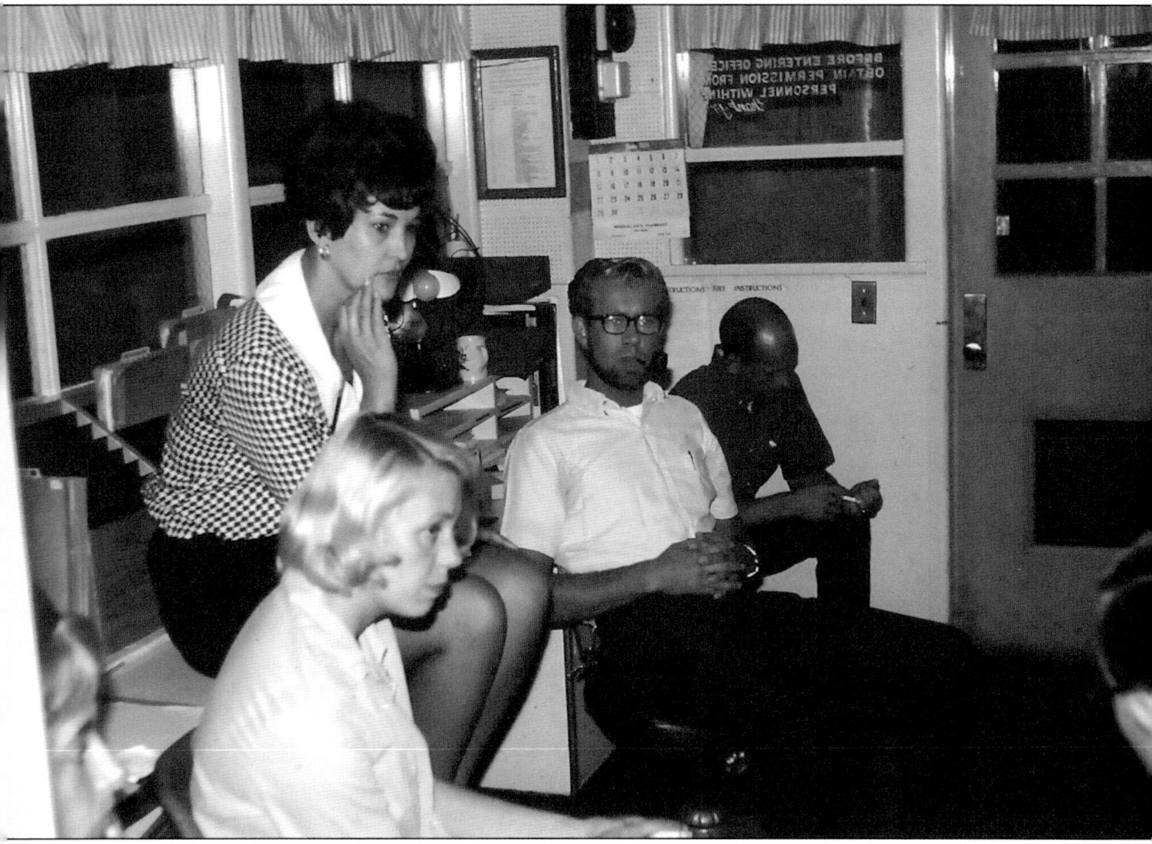

Staff met on a daily basis during shift changes to discuss their patients' progress. The patient population at Napa State Hospital peaked at 4,991 in 1960 and steadily declined as services for the mentally ill shifted to a community-based model. (Courtesy Peter Zwetsloot.)

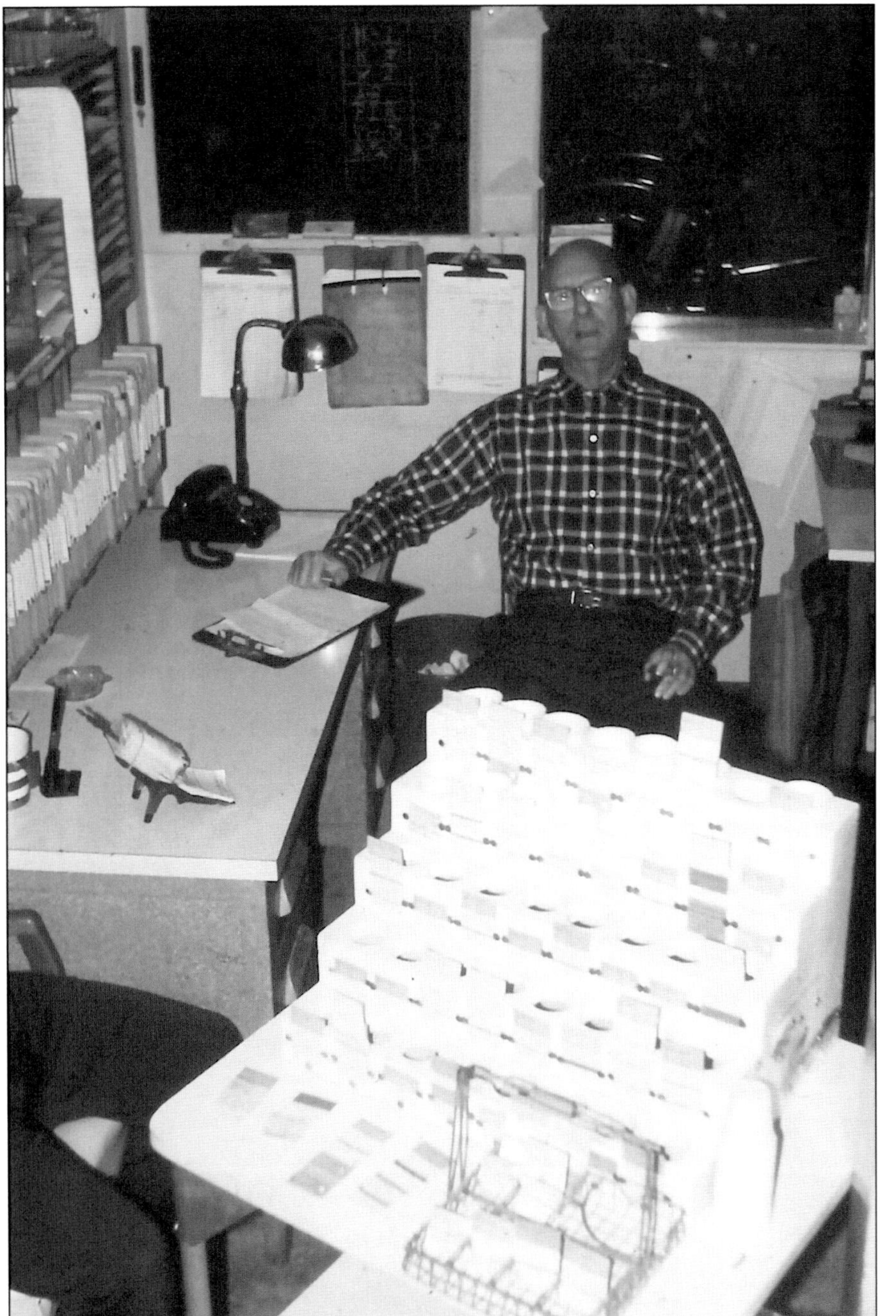

Breakthroughs in psychotropic drugs began during World War II when Valium was discovered to treat war veterans suffering from shell shock, or post-traumatic stress disorder. In 1946, the development of the antibiotic streptomycin effectively cured tuberculosis. Beginning in the 1950s, new drugs were used for treatment of epilepsy and syphilis. In the 1960s, as psychotropic drugs improved, patient populations in state hospitals began to decline. Psychosurgery, sterilization, and electroshock treatments were used less extensively, eliminating the need for surgical units. Pictured here is a psych tech. (Courtesy Peter Zwetsloot.)

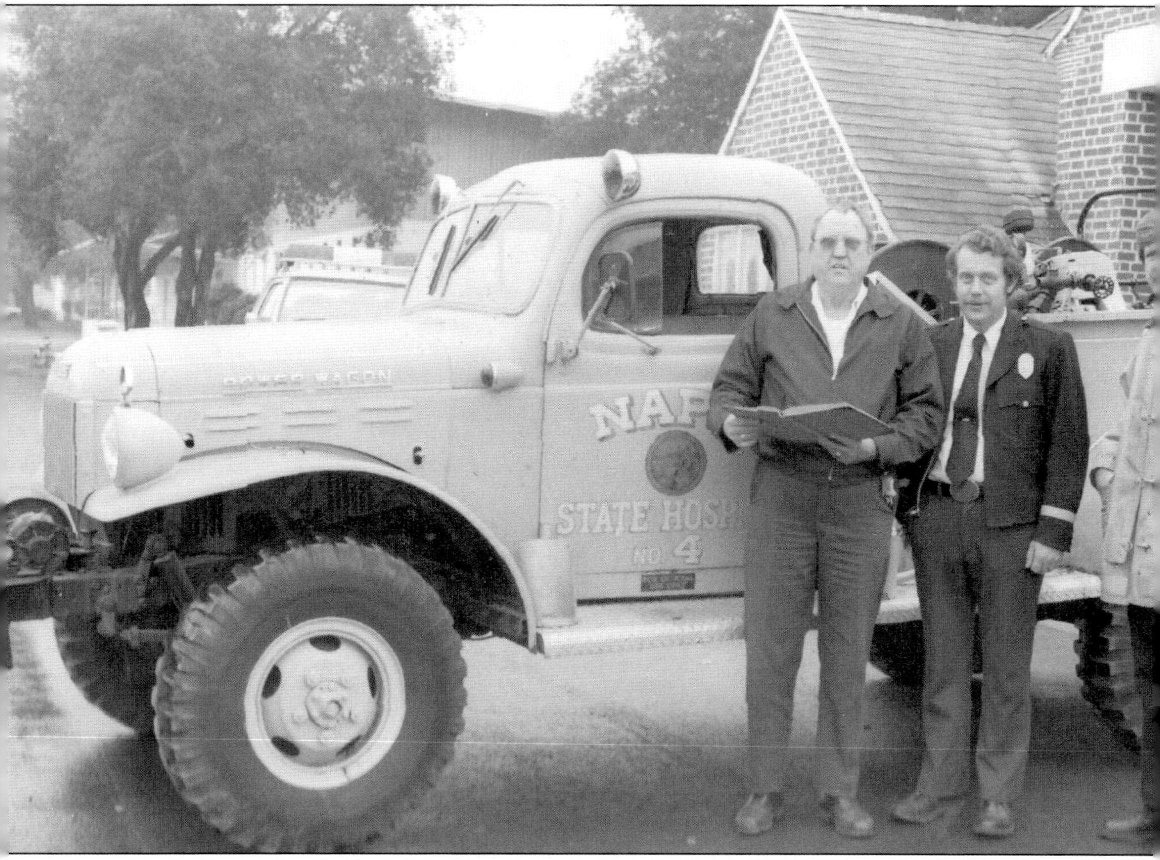

Vernon "Bud" Nowlin (left) is pictured with Pat Walmsley (center) and Ron Gupton. Each year, the patients and townspeople would line up to see Santa (Nowlin) on his sleigh as the fire chief towed him through the grounds. After 38 years of service, Bud retired shortly after this photograph was taken in the 1970s. His wife, Barbara Nowlin, was a psychiatric technician who went on to run the hospital's radio station, located in the receiving unit (B Ward), in the 1980s. (Courtesy Cindi Hummer.)

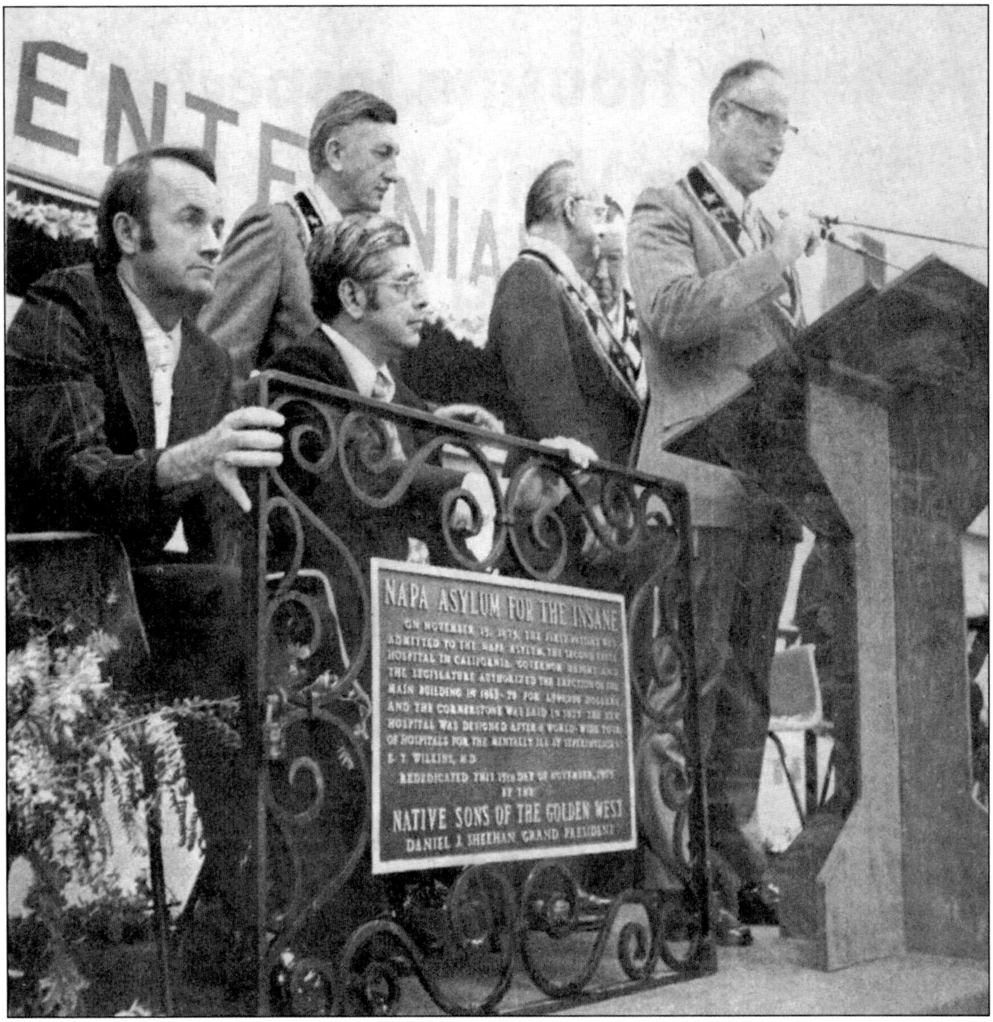

The Native Sons of the Golden West dedicated this plaque in a ceremony on November 17, 1975, celebrating Napa State Hospital's centennial. Controversy swirled around the plaque, which was titled "Napa Asylum for the Insane." Dr. Abraham S. Linn and Richard Friday are pictured here with Native Son grand president Daniel Sheehan at the podium. Interest in the history of the hospital was revived during preparations for the centennial celebration. Historian Ellen Brannick said, "The history committee's first meeting appropriately took place in an old hydrotherapy room in the Receiving [B] Ward." (Courtesy NCHS.)

Five

Postcard Perspectives

These postcards, having been widely distributed, are for some the only view of the Castle that was erected in 1875 and demolished in 1950. Most people in the United States, and especially in California, had never seen a building as grand as the Castle in the late 19th century. For 75 years it stood as a landmark: at times a source of pride and at others a symbol of the unpleasantness of asylum-keeping. Materials used in creating the grounds included 10 million bricks made on-site, 700,000 pressed bricks, 12,740 barrels of lime, 7,650 barrels of cement, 3,300 tons of slate roofing, and 1.5 million feet of lumber.

The original landscaping at the hospital was begun in 1880 under the direction of landscape architect J.D. Chalmers. One column, titled "A Revery," published in an 1882 edition of the *Asylum Appeal*, extols the beauty of the surroundings, "Who hath not loved at such an hour to drink in every breath? Violets, the faint, delicious, spring-time flower, kiss our feet. The cool soft grass is grateful to the touch. Green fields breathe sweet and leaf blossom, blade, hill, valley, the clear murmuring stream, mingle music with the strange deep harmonies that haunt my breast."

The administration building and new Receiving and Treatment Center, dedicated in 1954, represent an era of modest modernity in institutional buildings. It signified a return to complete focus on patient rehabilitation and reintroduction into the community.

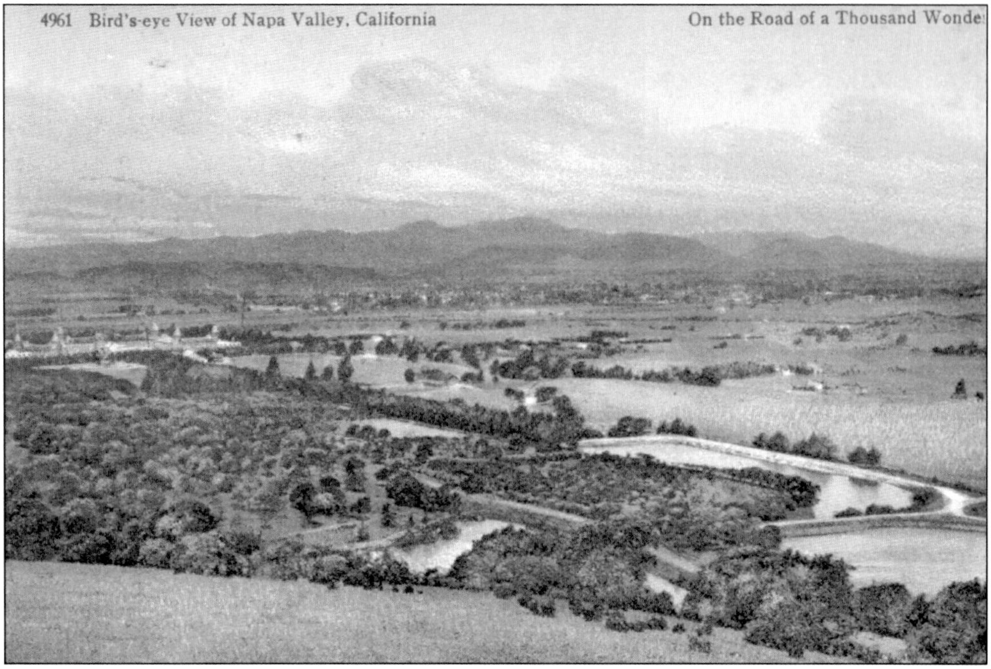
4961 Bird's-eye View of Napa Valley, California
On the Road of a Thousand Wonde

The Napa Valley and the Napa Asylum are pictured above in a 1890s postcard. The hospital is visible in the far upper left, and the Napa River landing is in the lower center, where supplies and patients were transported to Napa before being loaded onto horse-drawn carts and driven up Magnolia Drive and then a dirt road. A river scene is captured in the postcard below. (Courtesy Ellen Brannick.)

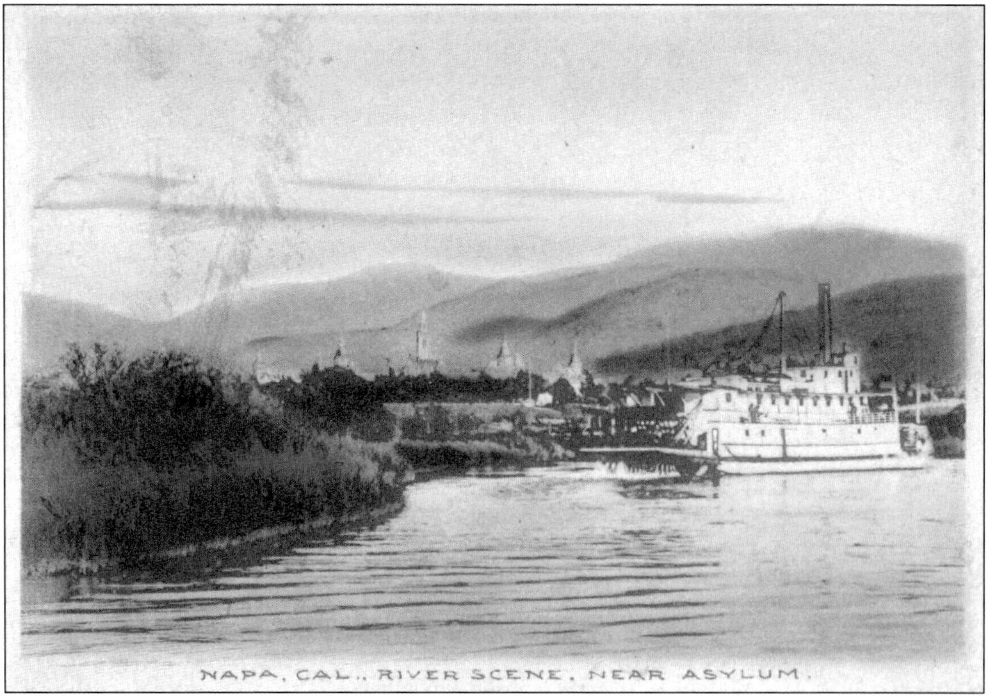
NAPA, CAL., RIVER SCENE, NEAR ASYLUM.

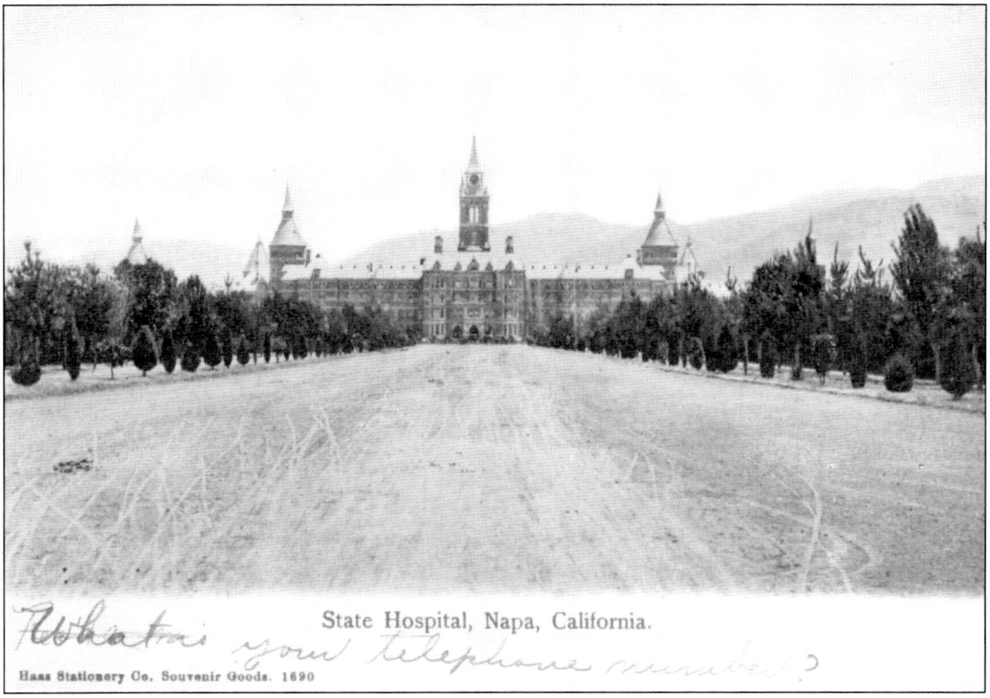

The initial property spanned 209 acres. It was enlarged to 2,062 acres over the years to accommodate water use, farming, and dairy operations. Many wards and units were locked to prevent disoriented patients from wandering off into town or, as is the case of one incident, into the nearby basalt quarry. By 1980, the grounds had been reduced to 1,500 acres. (Courtesy Todd Schulman.)

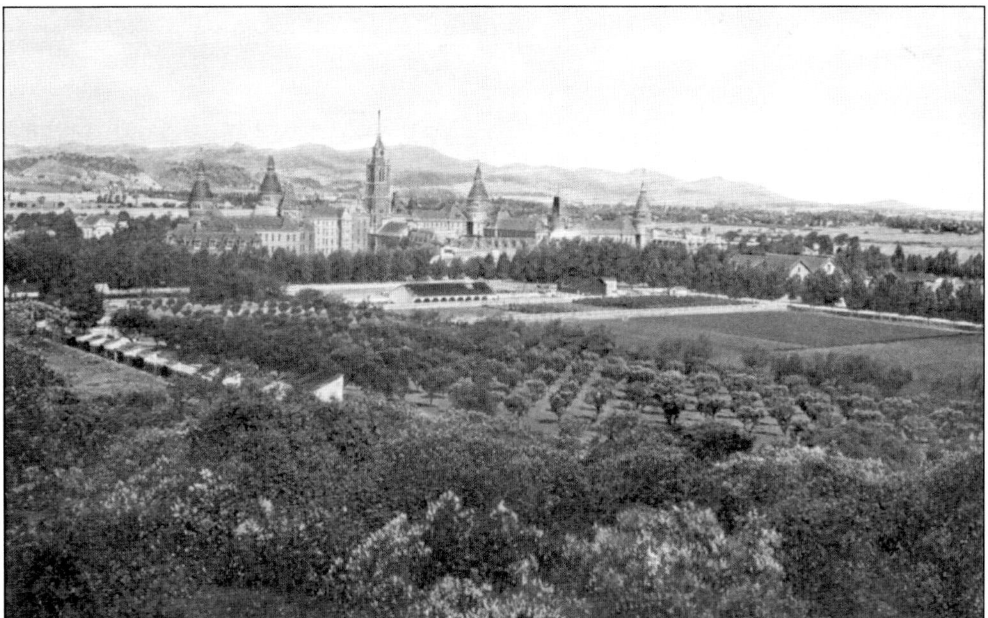

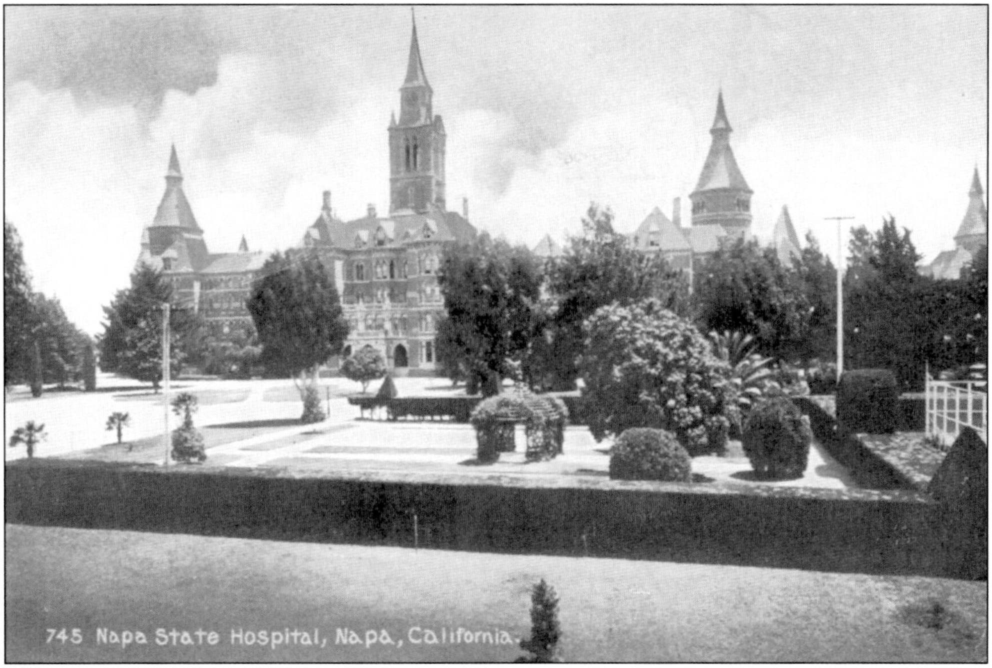
745 Napa State Hospital, Napa, California.

In his 1882 annual report, Dr. Edmund Wilkins expressed his gratitude to the state for providing an appropriation of funds for an additional water supply. In closing, he stated, "I thank God for the purity and abundance of this water, which has added so much to the comfort and safety of the Asylum, and to the beauty of the grounds. Green Lawns and beautiful shrubs, like the oasis in the desert, add their charms to the scene; while the sweet odors of lovely flowers perfume the air, and in silent eloquence express their praise. In the expressive language of Governor Perkins, when he saw the success of the enterprise, 'You have struck a bonanza!' and we are all happy with the result." (Courtesy Todd Schulman.)

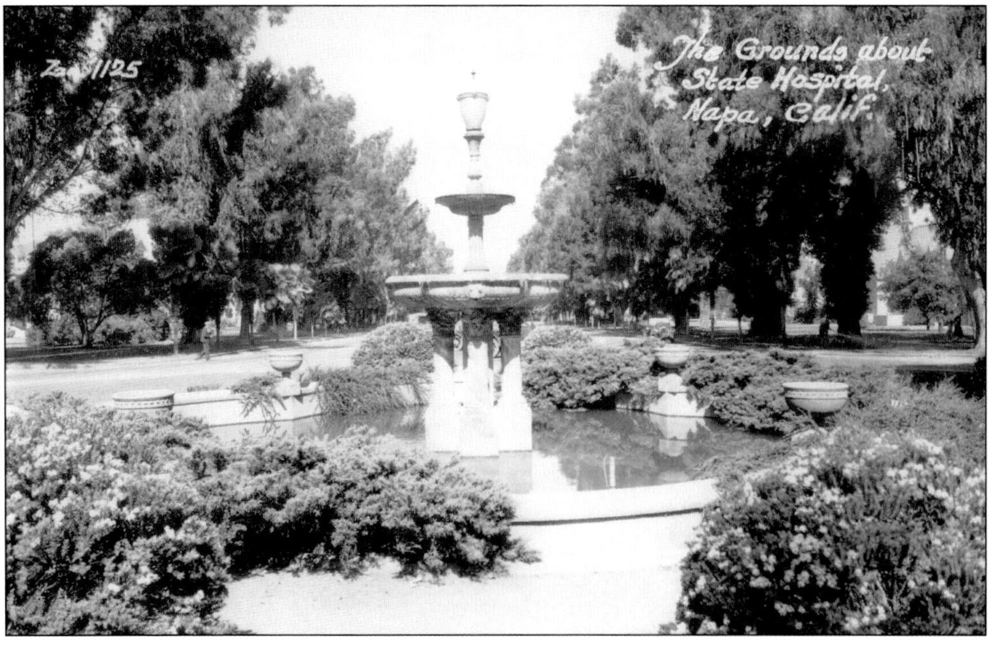
The Grounds about
State Hospital,
Napa, Calif.

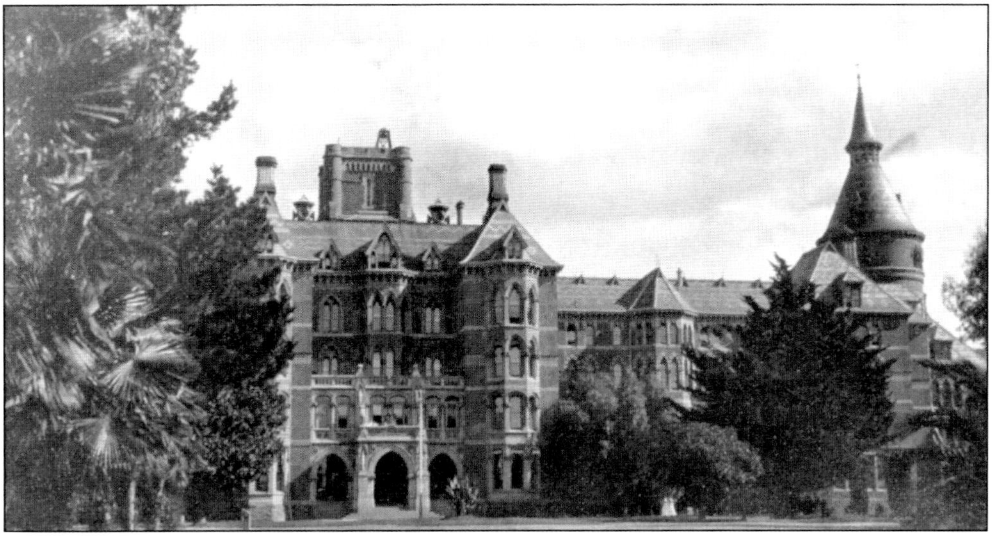

These two postcards, taken after the 1916 San Francisco earthquake, illustrate two stages of the process of lowering the main tower. (Courtesy Ellen Brannick.)

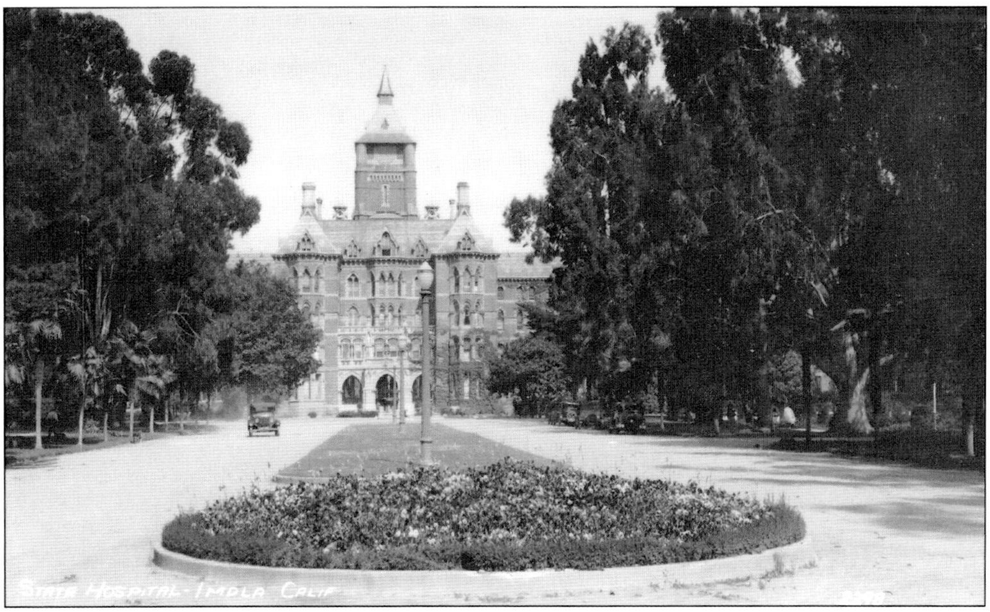

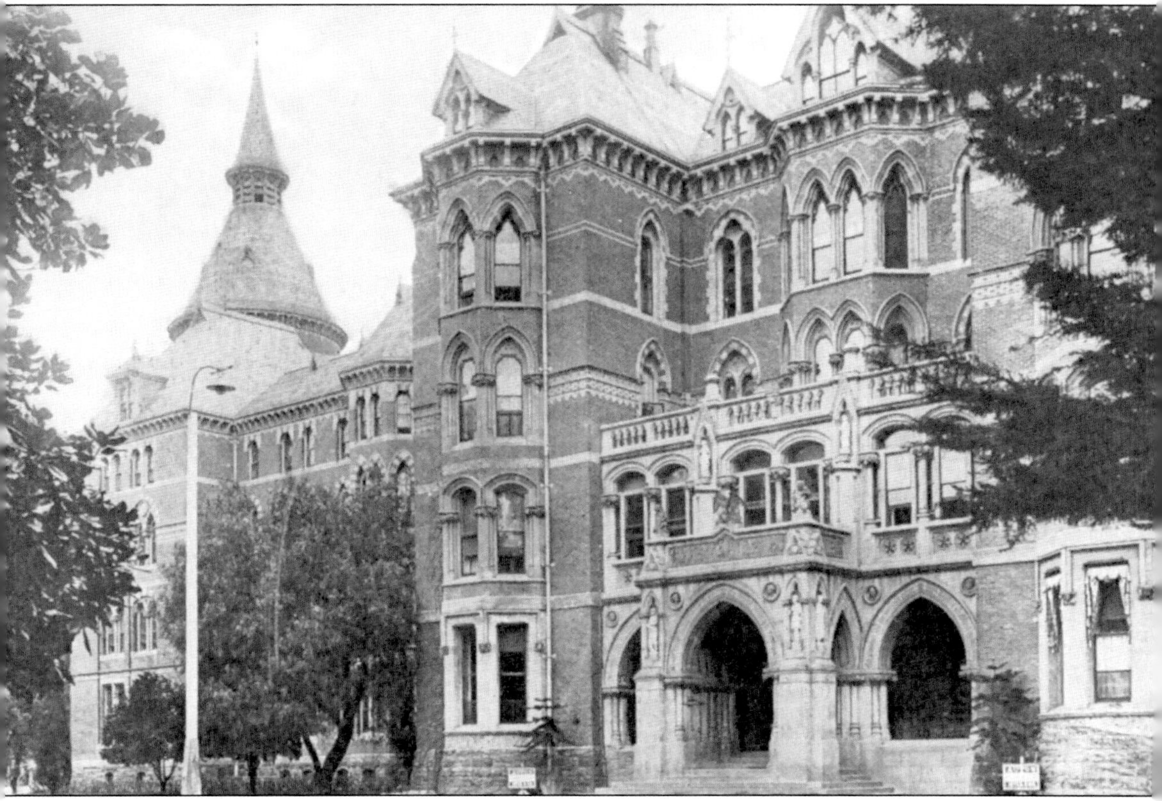

There are a number of theories as to why the Napa State Hospital was known as Imola. One states that the name was derived from a Native American word and another that the local postal clerk, who was from Italy, chose it because it reminded him of Imola, Italy, which also had an asylum. Most accounts lean toward the post office designation. (Courtesy Ellen Brannick.)

The postcard at left is labeled "Falls near State Hospital." It is actually Coombs Dam, which was one of the first structures built, in 1872, using stone from the quarry. The site was chosen because it was the narrowest point up South Tulocay Creek. The elevation provided the presser required for the water pipes leading to the building site. Coombs Dam was the only source for water until the Spencer Creek property was purchased in 1879. An ample water supply was essential to the hospital's operations, such as grazing areas for the dairy cows, shown below. (At right, courtesy Ellen Brannick; below, Todd Schulman.)

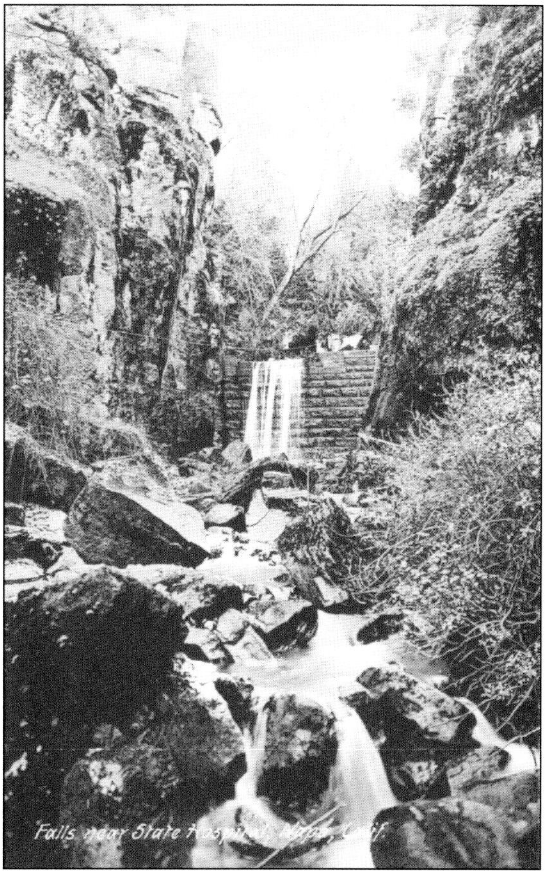

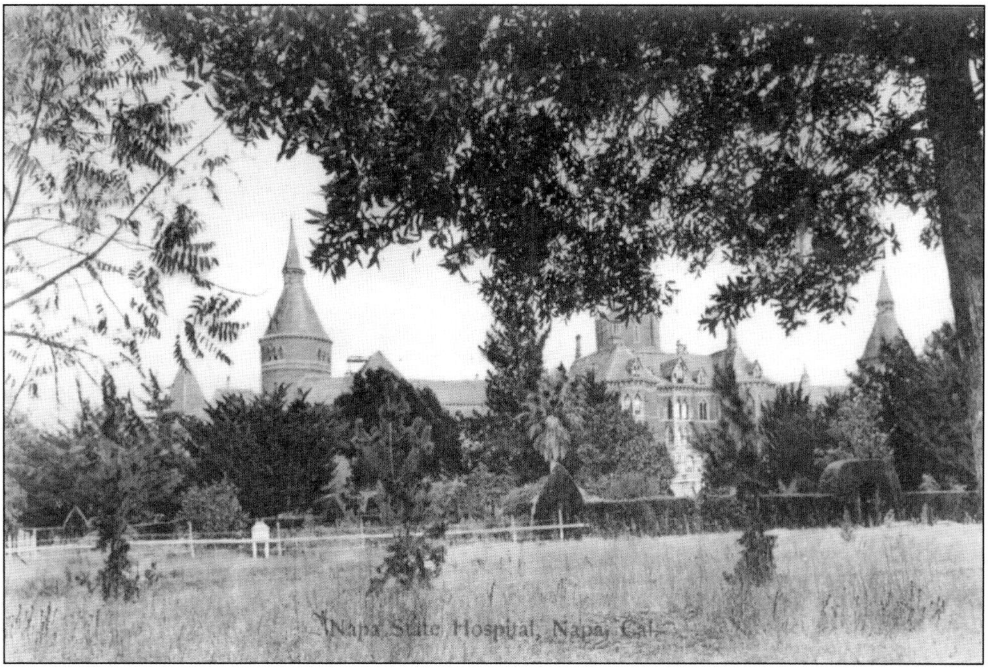

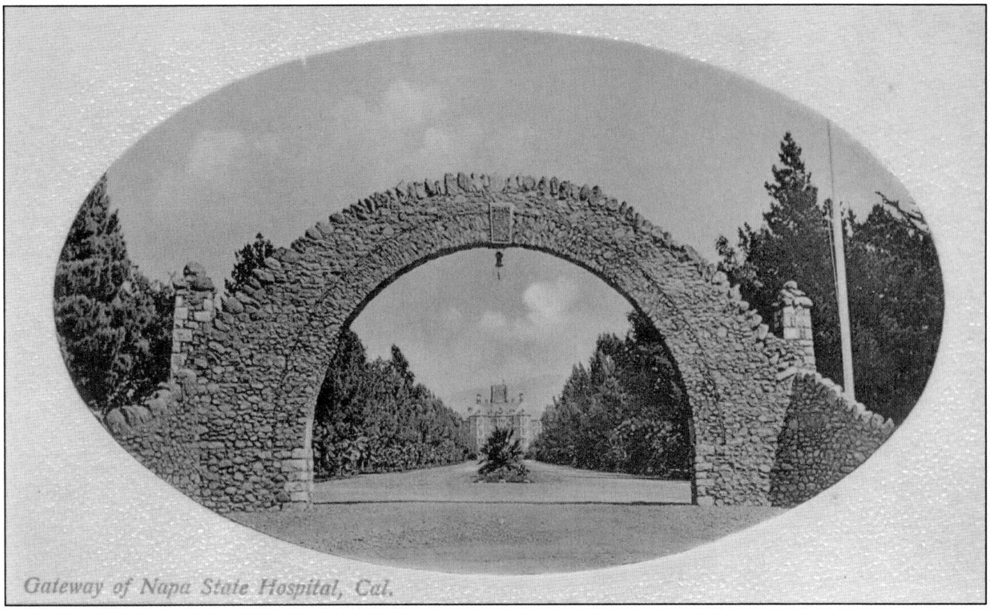

These two postcards, as well that on the following pages, illustrate the changing landscape and additional development of the property from the 1870s to the 1940s. Paved roads, additional landscaping, and a median were subsequently added. The original cornerstone was buried under one of the pillars of the gateway. (Courtesy Todd Schulman.)

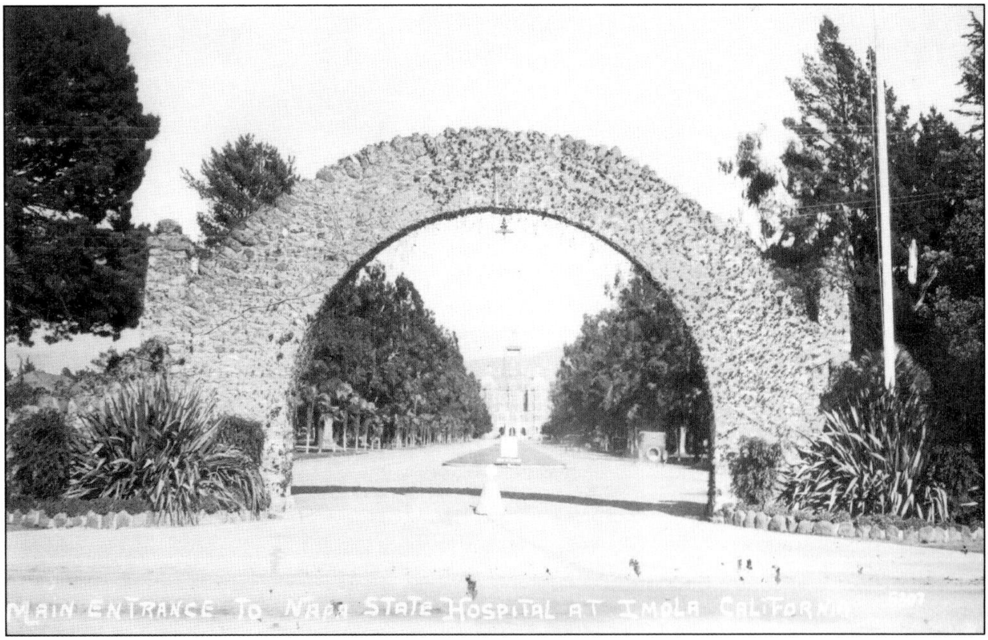

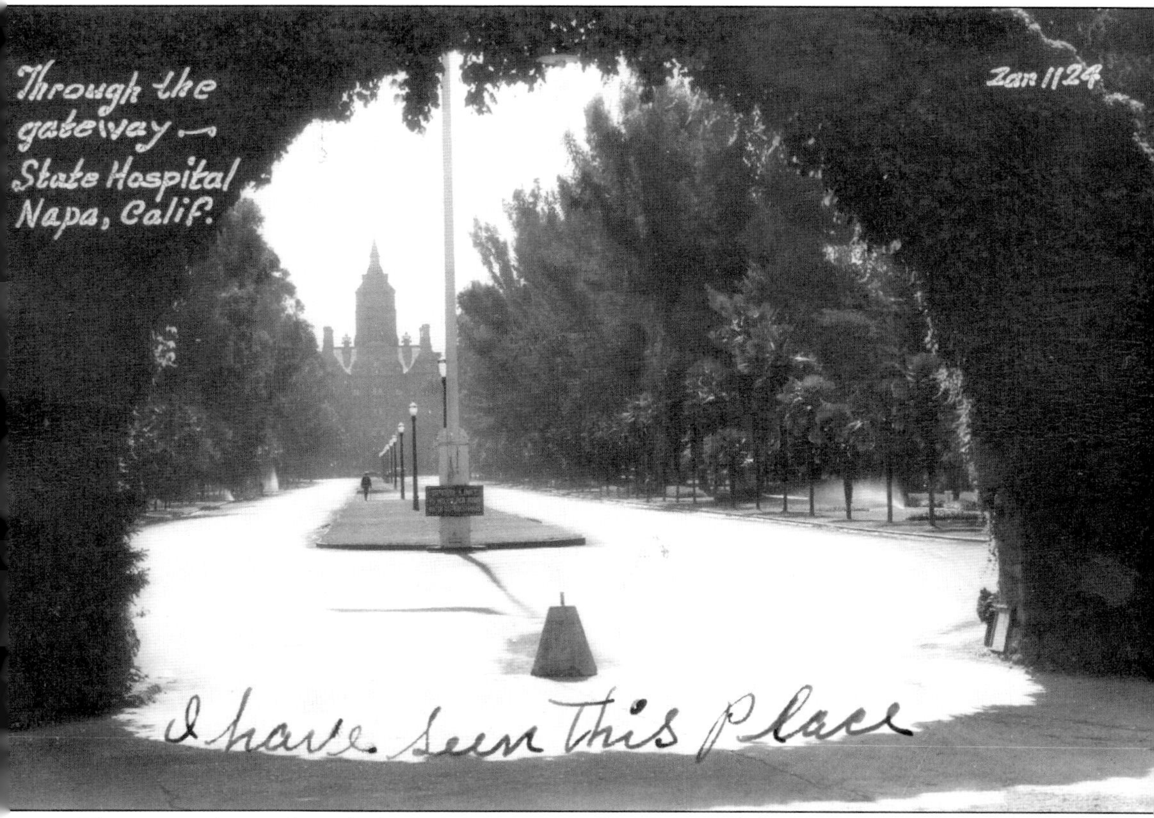
Through the
gateway —
State Hospital
Napa, Calif.
Zan 1124
I have seen this place

This postcard view through the gateway captures the serenity of Napa State Hospital. Note the sign: "Speed Limit 15 Miles per Hour. Watch for Pedestrians." (Courtesy Todd Schulman.)

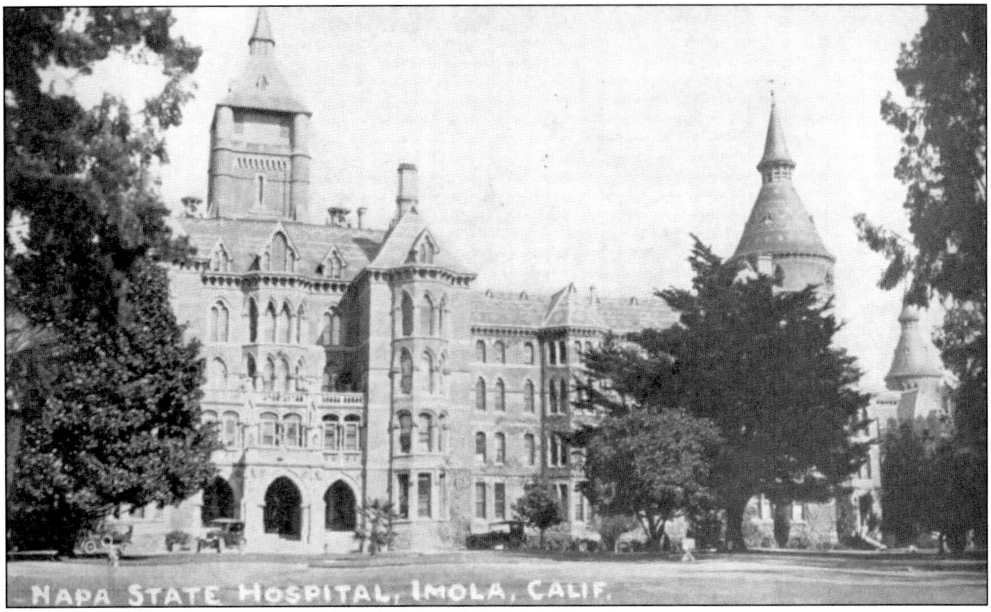

The Castle building was based on an improved Kirkbride Plan, which was introduced in the 1880 edition of *On the Construction, Organization, and General Arrangements of Hospitals for the Insane* by Philadelphia psychiatrist Thomas Story Kirkbride. The improved plan had a deeper V-shape, allowing for more separation between the wards, a fireproof staircase, specified alcoves or bay windows on the ends of ward hallways, and service buildings behind the central administration section. (Courtesy Todd Schulman.)

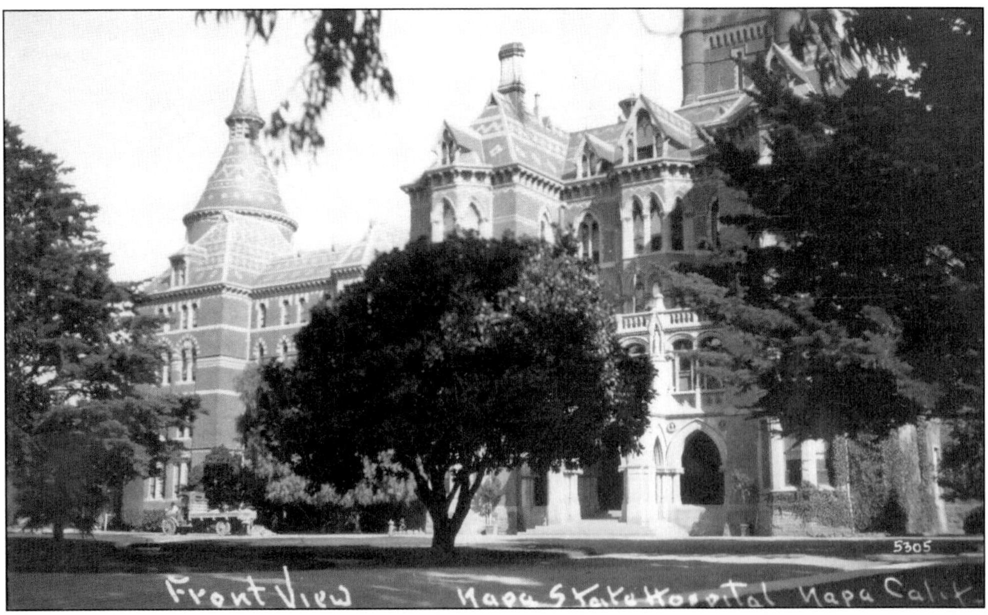

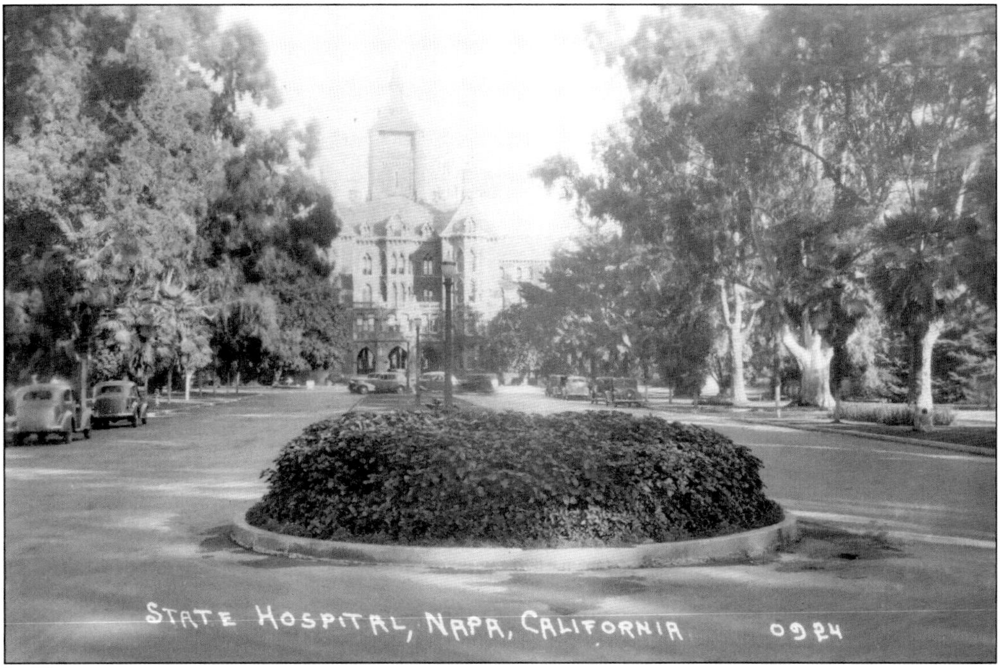

Contrasting views of the administration buildings in the 1940s (above), prior to demolition, and in the 1950s (below) illustrate the all-encompassing effort made to treat and house mentally ill and developmentally disabled patients. The state hospital system altered treatments, methodology, and staffing in order to meet the needs of rising patient populations, changing societal views on mental illness, and modern technology. (Above, courtesy Todd Schulman; below, Ellen Brannick.)

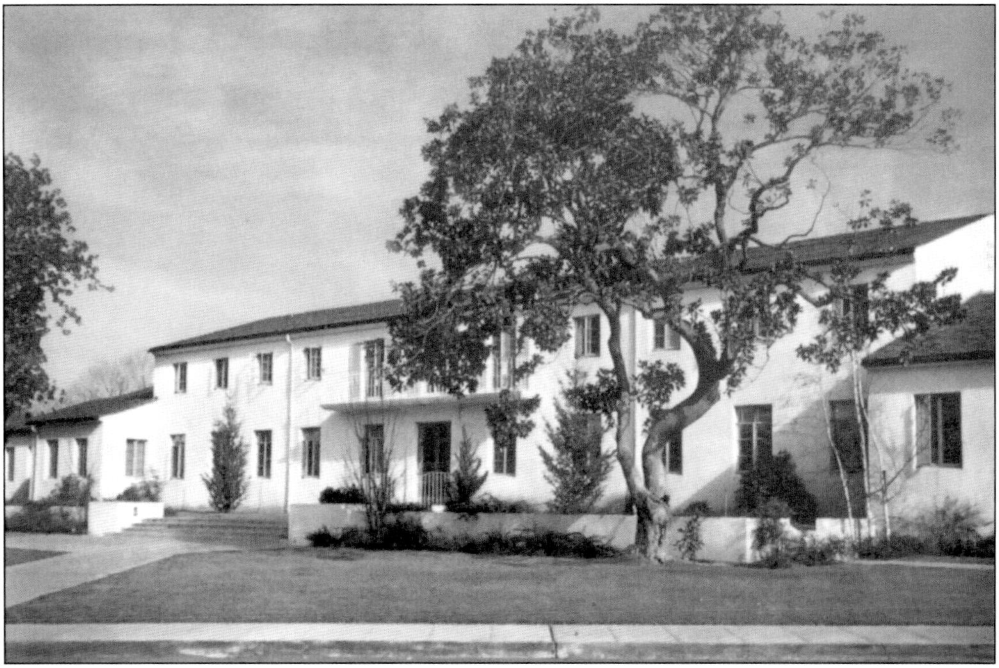